阴阳五行

朱宗元　原著

杨国英　张明锐　张立东　整理

蔡潇宇　翻译

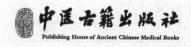

中医古籍出版社
Publishing House of Ancient Chinese Medical Books

图书在版编目（CIP）数据

阴阳五行/朱宗元原著；杨国英，张明锐，张立东整理；蔡潇宇翻译．–北京：中医古籍出版社，2019.12（2023.5重印）

ISBN 978 – 7 – 5152 – 1595 – 2

Ⅰ.①阴… Ⅱ.①朱…②杨…③张…④张…⑤蔡…

Ⅲ.①中医学–阴阳五行说 Ⅳ.①R22

中国版本图书馆 CIP 数据核字（2017）第 250051 号

阴阳五行

朱宗元　原著
杨国英　张明锐　张立东　整理
蔡潇宇　翻译

责任编辑　郑 蓉　英文编辑　秦 琳
封面设计　韩博玥
出版发行　中医古籍出版社
社　　址　北京市东城区东直门内南小街16号（100700）
电　　话　010 – 64089446(总编室)　010 – 64002949(发行部)
网　　址　www.zhongyiguji.com.cn
印　　刷　北京市泰锐印刷有限责任公司
开　　本　850mm×1168mm　1/32
印　　张　7.5
字　　数　160 千字
版　　次　2019 年 12 月第 1 版　2023 年 5 月第 4 次印刷
书　　号　ISBN 978 – 7 – 5152 – 1595 – 2
定　　价　30.00 元

前　言

历史悠久的中国医药学，有着独特的理论体系和丰富的实践经验。在当今世界医学之林中，闪耀着夺目的光彩。国内外学者越来越认识到中医学的珍贵蕴藏及对世界科学进步的深远影响。从而，现今形成了一股学习、研究中医学理论及文化的热潮。

阴阳五行学说，是中医学的重要理论基础，是中医学世界观和方法论形成中构建的核心元素。中医学的整体观、自然观都根植于此。然而，阴阳五行学说相对抽象，表述范围较为广博，且文理古奥、颇难索解。初学之人常感无从入手、叹为观止。为此，朱宗元先生在 1987 年撰写《阴阳五行学说》一书，以满足初学者之需求。该书较为详尽地阐述了阴阳五行学说的基本内涵，包括中医学的性质、中医学理论体系的形成、阴阳学说、五行学说等章节。该书可为初学中医的人员及广大中医爱好者了解与学习中医阴阳五行学说提供参考与借鉴。

内蒙古医科大学朱宗元教授，从事中医基础理论教学和研究几十年，他研读经典医著，师古而不拘经，择善而从，在研究和传承中医理论和文化方面精益求精，不断进取，具有独到见解，他经常向我们提起，如果这些理论能传播到国外，就会为中医学的发展作出更大的贡献。

在新时代人类生命科学发展的必然趋势和迫切需求下，我们在朱老师的鼓励和指导下，将他所著的《阴阳五行学说》予以修订并翻译成英文，面向国内外发行，以期增进中医学术的交流与传播。

全书所集资料丰富，说理深入浅出，例证翔实，倘能为探索医道披荆斩棘，鸣锣开道，则为所期，愿更好地为中医事业发挥应有的作用。

杨国英

目　　录

Contents

绪　言

中医学是世界上现存医学流派中最古老的医学之一，它的存在已有数千年的历史，是我国人民长期与疾病作斗争的丰富经验和结晶，是中华民族宝贵的文化遗产，也是东方文明的代表之一。在中医理论体系的形成过程中，它汲取了古代唯物论和辩证法思想，作为自己的指导思想和方法论，逐步形成了独特的医学理论体系，屹立于世界医林之中，为中国人民的保健事业和中华民族的繁荣昌盛作出了卓越的贡献。直到今天，中医学理论仍具有很大的科学价值，从而被世界医学界所重视。这就是我们今天仍要研究和发扬中医学的原因所在，并要使它在不久的将来，能为世界人民保健事业和生命科学的发展发挥更大的作用。

一、什么是"中医"

"中医"这一名称，大家都是非常熟悉的，但是进一步追究，似乎又不太明白。"中医"，实际上有两种涵义，我们不妨把它称为广义的"中医"和狭义的"中医"。

在古代，我国只有一种医学，那时并没有"中医"这个名称。随着西方医学传入我国，开始出现"洋医"这一名称，特别是鸦片战争以来，西方医学大量涌入我国，出现了两种医学并存的局面。为了区别这两种医学，和"洋医"相对应的出现了"国医"这个名称。"洋医"是指从西洋传入的医学，"国医"

1

是指我国固有的传统医学。大约近 70～80 年来，"洋医"又演变成"西医"，"国医"则演变成"中医"，这就是"中医"这个名称的由来。

"中医"既然是指我国固有的传统医学，它就应该包括所有起源于我国的各种传统医学，这就是广义"中医"所具有的涵义。

中国是一个多民族的国家，起源于中国的传统医学也不是只有一种，如起源于藏族集居地区的藏医，起源于蒙古民族集居地区的蒙医，其他还有维吾尔医、苗医、傣医等，它们都不同于起源于汉民族集居地区的汉医。就是起源于汉民族集居地区的还有草药医、蛇医等，也和汉医有明显的区别。广义的"中医"应包括所有起源于中国范围之内的传统医学，如汉医、藏医、蒙医、苗医、维吾尔医、傣医以及草药医、蛇医等。

在很多情况下，使用"中医"这个名称时，它不是包括我国所有的传统医学在内，而仅是指汉医。这是由于汉民族占我国人口的绝大多数，人口稠密，文化、经济发达的地区又多是汉民族集居的地区。起源于汉民族集居地区的汉医就成为我国绝大多数人口的传统保健方法，其在国内影响最大，而且还对国外产生一定的影响。另一方面，由于民族间的隔绝，其他民族医没有能在国内广泛流传，也不被占人口绝大多数的汉民族所了解。由于这些原因，自然地容易在"中医"和"汉医"之间划等号，而认为"汉医"就是"中医"，这样使用"中医"的概念，虽然不够确切，但却已成为习惯的用法。这就成为"中医"的第二种涵义，即狭义"中医"的涵义。

二、中医学的性质

（一）中医学属于传统医学的范畴

世界卫生组织将世界上现存的医学分为两大类：一为现代医学，一为传统医学。现代医学的形成是近 200～300 年的事，它是在西方传统医学的基础上，随着现代科学技术的发展而逐渐形成的，它是西方传统医学与现代科学技术相结合的产物。现代医学是以实验为依据，所以有人称它为"实验医学"。传统医学则有悠久的历史，它是随着人类的出现而逐渐形成的，是人类长期与疾病斗争的经验的积累。临床治疗经验的积累是传统医学发展的源泉，所以，传统医学又被称为"经验医学"。

中医学属于传统医学的范畴，是世界上现存传统医学中发展水平最高的，也是最大的一个医学流派。世界上现存的传统医学，多数仍停留在经验医学的阶段，如非洲、南美洲以及其他地区的传统医学，都是以丰富的医疗经验为医学的主体，加上有效的药物，构成了医学的主要部分。它们有丰富的治疗经验，对某些疾病的确有很好的疗效，但缺乏完善的理论。在医疗中，经验比理论更具有指导作用。中医学则不一样，虽然它也是以医疗经验为源泉，治疗经验在医疗中具有重要的作用，但它有一整套较完善的医学理论，这些理论对医疗的指导作用远远超过经验对医疗所起的作用。这说明中医学已从单纯的"经验医学"阶段上升到"理论医学"阶段。所以，中医学不同于一般的传统医学，而是具有高度理论水平的传统医学。

（二）中医学是"经验医学"和古代哲学的结合体

中医学之所以能够建立完善的医学理论体系，一是由于它在

3

开始形成之初，就和我国的古代哲学——阴阳五行学说相结合。并以这种朴素的唯物论和辩证法思想作为自己的指导思想和方法论，经过整理，把丰富的治疗经验提高到理性的高度，从而确立了独特的医学理论体系。二是因为中国历代政府对医学都比较重视，从周朝以下就形成了医官制度，开始分科，促进了医学向纵深发展。从南北朝以来，就建立了医学教育制度，促进了对医学理论的研究。而且历代几乎都由政府组织力量，对医药学进行总结和整理，编写了具有时代性的医学丛书、方书和药书，推动了中医学的发展。三是中华民族在传统上就比较重视医学，有不少思想家、科学家和军事家等都加入了医学研究的行列，用多种学科的知识来不断地充实医学理论，促使医学理论向纵深发展，并不断提高和完善。

在以上这些因素中，医学和古代哲学的结合，是中医学理论能达到高水平的关键因素。各学科知识向医学的渗透，不仅丰富了医学理论，促使中医学理论体系不断完善。而且能从认识论的角度上，保证指导思想的正确。因而中医学能建立一套具有较高水平并相当完善的理论体系。

（三）中医学的认识论

中医学不是建立在"实验医学"的基础之上的，但它是在"天人同理"思想的指导下，通过对天体、自然、社会和人体的大量观察，采用类比的方法，以自然、社会的规律或现象来认识人体和疾病，以整体的观点、运动的观点、辩证的观点来看待人体和疾病。中医学用宏观的、直观的和逻辑推理的方法，在活体的人身上来认识人体，从运动中来了解人体的组织结构和运动规律以及疾病的发生和发展规律，这种不同于现代医学的认识方法，某些方面甚至更优于现代医学，成为一种独特的医学理论体系。

中医学虽然有自己的优点，但也存在着缺点。中医学是用宏观的、直观的和逻辑推理的方法来认识人体和疾病，缺乏实验手段，在微观方面就显然不足了。因此，对人体和疾病的认识，在有些方面就缺乏一定的深度，甚至有的是错误的。此外，中医学的传统研究方法，主要是靠大量临床资料的积累。虽然这种研究方法曾经为中医学理论的形成和发展提供过大量的医学素材。但是，也不能不看到它的落后性和缺陷。从临床治疗中发现问题，总结规律，在医学形成的早期，是一种可取的方法，并能获得丰硕的成果。但是，当医学发展到今天，大量的医学规律都已被发现后，再采用以这种方法作为唯一的方法来发现问题，总结规律，其成功的机会是越来越少了，研究周期也越来越长，以至于在一个人的一生中也不可能完成必须的经验积累，而需要连续不断的几代人，甚至十几代人才能办得到。这正像在南京雨花台下乱石堆中寻找雨花石一样，在雨花石尚未出名前，寻石人不多，只要肯下功夫，花上半天、一天的时间，总能找到惟妙惟肖的雨花石。随着雨花石的名声增大，身价百倍，寻石者日益增多，雨花石却在减少。在这样的情况下再要去寻找雨花石，就必须花费更大的辛苦和更多的时间，有时还不一定能找到。正因为如此，中医学的流传研究方法就不再能适应医学发展的需要，反而成为导致中医学发展缓慢的主要原因。要改变这种状态，就必须改变研究方法和技术，缩短研究周期，提高工作效率，中医学才能加快发展。

中医学传统研究方法的另一个缺陷是单以临床疗效为依据，

这有很大的不可靠因素。临床疗效的取得受多种因素的影响，正确的治疗虽然是疾病痊愈的常见原因，但是，无效的治疗和疾病因其他原因而痊愈的巧合，在临床上也是屡见不鲜的。因此，单凭疾病痊愈就认为这位医生对疾病的认识是正确的，治疗是恰当的，这并不完全确切。由于这种原因，在中医理论中就不免掺杂一些不可靠因素。

每个医生的临床经验都是有一定的片面性的，以此总结出来的理论总是带有片面性。这是导致理论分歧的原因之一。再加上后人也无法进行重复，就无法对它进行肯定或否定，这样就使中医学理论中的"悬案"长期不决，后人难以适从。理论的"悬案"越多，中医文献就越是"浩如烟海"，这也是阻碍中医学理论发展的原因之一。

三、中医学理论体系的形成

中医学理论体系的形成，大约是在秦汉时期。它的形成过程也经历了数千年的时间，大致可以分成医学知识的积累、医学理论的萌芽和中医学理论体系的确立三个阶段。

（一）医学知识的积累阶段

医学是随着人类出现而开始逐渐形成的。人类最早的医疗活动，实际上是原始人类的自救本能。只有在人类为了生存与繁衍后代，通过劳动促进了人类大脑的进化和智力发展以后，原始人类自救本能的医疗活动，才开始转变为一种知识，并积累成为医疗经验。医疗经验的积累，加深了人类对疾病的认识，使人类的医学知识不断丰富，成为医学理论的素材。

医学知识的积累经过了漫长的时间，春秋（公元前770年）

6

以前都属于这一阶段。远古人类的医疗活动并无文字记载，只是后人根据传说记载于史书之中而流传下来。根据西晋·皇甫谧《帝王世纪》的记载，我国传说中的人类的始祖、渔猎畜牧的创导者——伏羲氏制作了"八卦"，用来说明疾病发生的机理，是传说中的中医学理论的创始者。传说他还发明了"九针"（包括各种类型针刺用针和脓肿切开手术等九种医疗器具）。西汉人所著的《纬礼》记载了我国传说中火的发现者——燧人氏钻木取火，教导人们吃熟食，避免胃肠道疾病的发生。根据西汉·淮南王刘安所著《淮南子》的记载，我国传说中农业和医药的发明者神农氏为了寻找药物，亲自尝试药物，有时一天之中能发生七十次中毒反应。西晋·皇甫谧的《针灸甲乙经》记载，传说我国中原地区的帝王——黄帝为了探求医理，和他的臣子岐伯、少俞、伯高等人，经常讨论人体的解剖和生理知识，探讨医学的理论，阐明了针灸学的道理。这些传说不一定完全真实，但它所说的故事，反映了我国远古的人民曾为医学的形成、医学知识的积累作出过重大贡献，付出了辛勤的劳动，这是不容怀疑的。

相传在夏代（公元前 21 世纪—公元前 16 世纪）我国已开始了酿酒。《战国策》有仪狄作酒进献夏禹的记载。酒的出现，医生用酒治病，曾经是一种重要的治疗方法，促进了医学的发展。

到了殷商时期（公元前 16 世纪—公元前 11 世纪），医学知识有了进一步积累，对疾病的认识也有加深。根据甲骨文的记载，在武丁时期（公元前 1324 年—公元前 1266 年），绝大多数疾病是按发病的部位笼统记载，如疾首（头病）、疾目（眼病）、疾耳（耳病）、疾身（腹病）等。这说明当时对人体部位的划分已经明确，但对疾病的症状只有模糊而笼统的印象。而少数疾病则有特定的名称，如疟、疥、蛊、龋等。说明当时对这些疾病的主要特征已有一定的了解。这时认为疾病是由于冒犯了祖先，祖先给予惩罚所致。因此在治疗上，主要是采用祈祷和祭祀，以求祖先的宽恕。这时期也认识到饮食、气候、环境和疾病的发生有一定的关系，并认识到舞蹈可以增强体质，能预防和治疗某些疾病。

西周时期（公元前 11 世纪—公元前 770 年）医学知识仍在缓慢地积累，人们对疾病的认识有了明显地加深。《山海经》记载的 38 种疾病中，有 23 种是根据疾病的主要特征来命名的，如瘕疾、疥、瘅、疣、疽、痹、瘘、蝎、瘿、疬、疟、狂、痔等；有 12 种是按症状命名，如肿疾、聋、咽痛、心痛、呕等；以部位表示病名的只有 3 种，如腹病、心腹之病等。这和武丁时期比较已有明显的进步。《山海经》还记载了 120 种药物，多数为植物药和动物药，其他还有矿物药等。这一时期虽然祈祷和祭祀仍然是治疗的主要方法，但是，药物疗法已有重大的发展。

在这一时期，除了医学知识进行积累、治疗方法得到发展外，和中医学理论有关的阴阳学说、五行学说也在孕育之中。传说中的伏羲氏制"八卦"，再经周文王推演而成"六十四卦"，就是对相反相成、对立统一规律的演绎。这一时期"阴阳"和"五行"的概念均在萌芽之中，从对日的向背引出了"阴阳"，从日常生活必不可少的因素中概括出"五材"，为"五行"概念的形成准备了条件。

（二）医学理论的萌芽阶段

春秋时期（公元前 770—公元前 476 年），是医学理论的萌芽阶段，一是作为中医学理论基础的古代哲学理论体系的发展，二是医学知识的积累已开始向理论过渡，中医学理论的某些基本观点已有雏形。

春秋时期是我国奴隶制社会向封建社会过渡的转变时期，新兴地主阶级的出现，提出了变革的要求，产生了新的学术思想。诸子百家，蜂拥而起，学术气氛出现了空前活跃的盛况。具有朴素唯物主义和辩证法思想的阴阳学说、五行学说也得到了较大的发展，其理论体系在逐步形成，并被广泛地应用于解释各种自然及社会现象。

"阴阳"是我国古代人民在生活及劳动中逐渐形成的概念，最初仅是就太阳的向背而言。《段注说文》说："阴，水之南，山之北；阳，高明也。"注："水南山北，日所难及。"古人是把向着太阳的一面或地高易被太阳照射之处称为"阳"，而把太阳照不到的低洼地区称为"阴"。在这些基础上，逐渐就把"阴阳"作为事物内部对立统一双方的代表，成为具有普遍意义的抽象概念，而不再是指具体的事物或现象。根据《国语》记载，西周幽王二年（公元前 780 年）西周三川发生了地震，伯阳父认为"阳伏而不能出，阴迫而不能蒸，于是有地震"。伯阳父用阴阳失去平衡来解释地震的发生，阳气潜伏而不能出，阴气迫于内而得不到蒸化，当蕴结到一定程度，突然暴发出来，于是就发生了地震。《周易》认为"一阴一阳谓之道"。即是认为"阴阳"是自然界的普遍规律。这一时期阴阳学说已有了雏形，一是认为"阴阳"是自然界的普遍规律；二是把"阴阳交感"当作是自然界万物生长变化发生的原因；三是建立了"阴阳平衡"的概念，用"阴阳失调"（即阴阳失去平衡）来解释异常现象的发生。

"五行"的概念最初是我国古代人民从生活和劳动中概括出来的,是人们生活及劳动所不可缺少的,最早称为"五材"。而后又把它们当成是构成万物的基本物质,即有某种程度的"元素"的含义。进一步又把木、火、土、金、水的属性抽出来,而成为只表示五种属性的抽象概念,这样,"五行"就成为一种哲学概念,不再是指具体的物质。"五行"作为一种抽象的概念,并认为任何事物或现象的内部都包含有这五种属性。因此,就把用来解释自然及社会现象的"五行",引入医学之中。这一时期,五行学说正处在形成之中,一是"五行"的概念已被抽象化;二是"五行"已被当作自然规律来应用,"五行"间的平衡和协调是事物存在和发生发展的必要条件;三是"五行"间关系的破坏,是事物发生异常变化的主要原因。

老子即老聃,大约生于周简王六年(公元前580年),约卒于周敬王二十年(公元前500年),是春秋末期人物。老子著《老子》(后来被称为《道德经》)一书,一是提出"道"是世界的核心,为万物之源,为"气"或"精气"学说的先声;二是提出了"无为"的思想,认为人当顺应自然,不可求者不当强求,中医学中"养生"学说和"效法自然"的思想深受《老子》的影响;三是书中充满了辩证法思想,《老子》的辩证法思想对中医学理论体系产生了重要的影响。

春秋时期,奴隶制瓦解,封建地主阶级兴起,尤其是在春秋后期,周室王权日益削弱,诸侯的权势日趋增强,神权也随之衰落,在医学方面就反映在鬼神致病也被人们所怀疑。如郑国子产就认为,疾病是"出入饮食哀乐之事也,山川星辰之神又何与焉?"（疾病是由出入＜生活行为＞、饮食、哀乐＜情志因素＞所引起的，和山川星辰之神又有什么关系呢？）齐国的晏婴也认为，疾病是"纵欲厌私"的结果。根据《左传》记载，周景王四年（公元前451年）秦国的医和给晋平公诊病，他说："天有六气，降生五味，发为五色，徵为五声，淫生六气。六气曰阴、阳、风、雨、晦、明也。分为四时，序为五节，过则为菑；阴淫寒疾，阳淫热疾，风淫末疾，雨淫腹疾，晦淫惑疾，明淫心疾。"从这段议论中可以看出，春秋末期及战国初期，医学理论已处于萌芽阶段，已形成了一些基本观点：一是把疾病的病因和自然、社会等因素联系起来，认为气候、环境、生活习惯、情志、饮食、房室等因素过度，即能发生致病作用，和神鬼无关；二是把"天人相应"的观点引入医学，作为医学理论的基本观点之一；三是把"阴阳"的概念引入医学，提出"阴淫寒疾，阳淫热疾"是《内经》"阴盛则寒""阳盛则热"的起源，"风淫末疾、雨淫腹疾"和后世对风邪、湿邪的认识也是一脉相承的；四是把五行的概念引入医学，提出了五味、五色、五声、五节以及四时、六气的概念，实为《内经》相关理论奠定了基础。

经过了春秋时期，与医学有关的古代哲学理论逐渐完善，医学知识的积累已开始向医学理论升华，这就为中医学理论体系的形成准备了充分的条件。

（三）中医学理论体系的形成

中医学理论体系的形成，大约开始于战国时期（公元前476—公元前221年），一直到东汉（公元25—220年）末年或三国时期（公元220—265年）才完成。它是以《黄帝内经》《神农本草经》和《伤寒杂病论》三书的成书为标志。在这一时期内，一是作为中医学理论的基石——古代哲学理论的完善，二是中医学理论体系的形成，从而使中医学理论体系得到确立。

1. 中医学理论的基石——古代哲学理论的完善

盖房屋要打地基，基础打得好坏，直接影响房屋的质量。基础不牢固，房屋盖得再好，寿命也不会长久。中医学理论体系有自己的基础，它的基础就是长期取得的丰富的治疗经验和医学知识。同理，其他国家或地区的传统医学也都是建立在这个基础之上的。但是，当现代医学兴起后，多数传统医学都处于消亡状态。唯独中医学仍有所发展，关键在于中医学在其理论体系形成之初，就吸取了正确的古代哲学作为自己的指导思想和方法论。它充分地运用了古代哲学的观点和方法，对丰富的治疗经验和医学知识进行了综合分析，演绎推理，使它成为层次分明、纲目清晰、系统而完整的医学理论体系，中医学理论体系也就因此而确立。和中医学理论关系最密切的古代哲学思想有阴阳学说、五行学说和精气学说。

阴阳学说在春秋时期已初步形成，到战国时期又有了进一步的发展。由于"阴阳"概念的抽象化，因而得到了广泛的应用。任何事物或现象都可以分为"阴阳"两个组成部分，就是形成宇宙的原始物质——"气"，也可以分为"阴阳"二气。其清轻者为"阳"，上升以成为天；其重浊者为"阴"，下降以成为地。进一步又用"阴阳"对立统一的关系、"阴阳"运动变化的规律、"阴阳平衡"的概念来解释自然及社会现象，"阴阳"就成为自然界运动变化的根本规律。

对于自然界中普遍存在着相反相成、对立统一的现象，我国古代早有认识。传说中的"伏羲氏制八卦"就是对相反相成、对立统一普遍性的概括。相传"周文王演八卦",推演为"六十四卦",而著《易经》。《易经》用"—"爻和"——"爻来表示相反相成、对立统一的双方,进行了推演,包含有很多的辩证法思想。在战国时期成书的《易传》,就把"—"爻直接称之为"阳",把"——"爻称之为"阴",这样就把阴阳学说和"八卦"理论合为一体,使阴阳学说中的辩证法思想得到进一步的充实,阴阳学说也才成为更为完善的哲学理论。

"五行"最早被称为"五材"或"六府"("六府"比"五材"多一个"谷",说明当时一部分学者非常强调"民以食为天"。而"五材"把"谷"归属于"木"中),后来"五行"的概念被抽象,并且为了更进一步强调"五行"之间的联系方式和它运动变化的属性,所以采用"五行"的名称,而未用"五材"或"六府"的叫法。

"五行"间的联系方式,即"五行"的"相生"和"相胜"的关系。"五行相胜"的概念形成得比较早,《墨子》已有"五行无常胜"的提法,说明"五行相胜"的概念早已存在。但在"相胜"是否有固定的顺序,是有争论的。"五行相胜"的顺序,大约到战国的后期由邹衍(公元前340—公元前260年)确定的。根据《文选·魏都赋注》引《七略》的解释和《吕氏春秋·应同篇》的记载,邹衍创造的"五德终始"的学说就是按"五行相胜"的顺序进行的。关于"五行相生"的顺序,先秦诸子著作并未提及,只是从"五行"和"五时"相配的顺序来看,可能在战国时期已经形成了。"五行相生"和"相胜"的顺序主要是根据对自然现象的观察中得出来的。虽然"五行相生"和"相胜"的本身并没有反映事物的本质联系，但用"相生"和"相胜"的方式来说明事物间的联系方式，特别是建立了"五行生克"的基本模式，确能反映事物间相互联系的一般性规律，具有很大的科学价值。

五行学说是有特殊意义的，除建立了"五行生克"模式以外，另一方面表现在"五行"和"数"的关系。在我国古代对"数"就有较深刻的认识，如《左传》说："物生有两、有三、有五……故天有三辰，地有五行。"《国语》也说："天六地五，数之常也。"在这个认识过程中，二是一个关口，"阴阳"就是以二为基数的"二分法"。五也是一个关口，"五行"则是以"五"为基数的"五分法"。在自然界与社会中，事物间的相互关系，归结起来只有"利"和"害"两种关系，以"五"为基数建立起来的模式是表示这两种关系的最基本模式。任何大于或小于"五"而建立起来的模式，都不能构成表示这两种关系的最简明的基本模式。

精气学说原是道家的理论，是用来解释世界的起源和统一性的。精气学说被引入了医学之后，即成为中医学理论的基石。

道家创始人老子认为"道"是世界的核心，它在物质世界形成之前已经存在，世界万物都是起源于"道"。《庄子》认为世界万物起源于"气"，把"道"解释为"气"。《公羊传》又提出"元气"为天地之始。到了战国的末期，宋鈃、尹文又提出了"精气"的概念，他们认为"精气"是气之精粹部分，是万物的本源。并明确地把"道"解释为"气"。"气"是客观世

14

界的本身，是无处不有的。世界上一切有形的物体都是由"气"所构成的。"精气"又是任何生命物质所不可缺少的，人体同样是由"精气"结合而成的。"精气"的流行变化则产生了生命现象、精神意识和思维活动。其后荀子又提出了"形具而神生"的命题，进一步肯定了精神是形体的产物，精神是不能离开形体而单独存在的。就这样，精气学说实际上是开始于春秋末期的老子，到了战国的末期已形成了自己的理论体系，肯定了"气"或"精气"的物质性是构成世界万物的本源，也是生命体的本源；也确定了生命现象、精神意识都是形体的产物，是"气"或"精气"运动的表现。

到了战国末期的邹衍，在精气学说的基础上，把精气学说、阴阳学说和五行学说三者揉为一体，加以系统化，而形成了"阴阳五行学说"，成为一个独立的理论体系。《黄帝内经》在总结前人医疗经验、医学理论时，正是采用了以精气学说为基础的"阴阳五行学说"作为医学理论的基石和指导思想，创立了自己的理论体系，从而奠定了中医学的理论基础。

2.《黄帝内经》是中医学的理论体系基本确立的标志

《黄帝内经》（简称《内经》）是现存最早的一部中医理论专著，在《汉书·艺文志》中已有记载，说明《内经》在西汉末年以前已经成书。它可能是根据春秋战国以来的医学理论著作，摘其精要者编汇而成的。所以内容庞杂，前后不一，甚至有自相矛盾之处。今日所见之《内经》又屡经后人传抄、删改和增补，和原来面貌已不完全一样，但在主要内容上、理论体系上没有重大的变化。

现存的《内经》包括《素问》和《灵枢》(《灵枢》又名《针经》)两部，各9卷81篇，共18卷162篇。长期流传，原书散佚不全。唐·王冰重新编注时，《素问》已缺9篇，后找到《天元纪》《五运行》《六微旨》《气交变》《五常政》《六元正纪》《至真要》等7篇大论补入，但仍缺《刺法》《本病》二论。故在王冰编注时，《素问》实存79篇。北宋·高保衡等人校正医书时，《灵枢》残缺过甚而无法校正，仅校正了《素问》。高氏当时又发现了《刺法》与《本病》二论，但和《素问》其他各篇比较，有显著的不同，故未被高氏收入《素问》，后人则将此二篇编成《素问遗篇》。到宋哲宗八年(公元1093年)高丽献书中有一部完整的《针经》，自此国内重新见到完整的《针经》，即今所见的《灵枢》。

《内经》是一部医学理论专著，内容涉及广泛，但是仍以医学基础理论为中心议题。它在医学上的贡献是确立了中医学的医学理论体系，它的主要观点如下：

(1) 继承了"气——元论"的思想 "气——元论"是我国古代朴素的唯物主义思想的基本观点，它认为"气"是万物之本源，万物之间的差异是由于"气"运动形式的不同而引起的。《内经》继承了这一观点，认为世界是由于"气"的运动而产生的，"气"充实于整个宇宙之中，在不停地运动着。正是由于"气"的不断运动，才引起了四季的更替、万物的更新和传代、生命体的生和亡的交替。人也是由"气"所构成的，人就是依靠"气"的运动来维持正常的生命活动，"气"运动的失常，正常生命活动不能维持，就要引起疾病的发生以致死亡，所以《素问·举痛论》说："百病生于气也"。

由于世界是由"气"构成的，人也是由"气"所构成的；由于"气"的运动，引起了自然界的变化，也引起了人的生命活动，"气"就成为人和自然界统一的物质基础。也就成为"天人相应"理论的根据了。

（2）确立了整体观念 《内经》所确立的整体观念有两方面的涵义，一是"天人一体观"，二是人的整体性原则。

"天人一体观"，是说天（即自然界、整个宇宙）和人是存在于一个整体之中，人是自然界的组成部分之一。它又包含两重意思，一是"天人相应"，二是"天人同理"。

"天人相应"，即是说人和自然界的结构是相似的，人是自然界的一个缩影。因此，自然界有的结构，在人体身上就有相应的结构；自然界发生的任何变化，都要在人体上引起相应的反应。所以《灵枢·岁论》说："人与天地相参也，与日月相应也。"例如一年有四季的变化，在植物中就要引起春生（萌芽）、夏长（生长）、秋收（开花结果）、冬藏（枯萎）的变化。在人体上也随季节发生相应的变化，春夏生长力旺盛，秋冬生长力相应的减弱。另外，每当节气交替或气候变化的时候，有不少慢性疾病（尤其是腰腿痛之类的疾病）都要发病，这就是气候变化引起人体发生相应的反应。

"天人同理"是说明自然界的变化和人体的变化有共同的或类似的规律性。根据这一理论，就可以引用自然界发生变化的规律性来解释人体发生的相似变化。如风能引起自然界出现"动"的现象，如树枝的摇动，甚至还可以引起飞沙走石；那么在人身体上出现"动"的症状，如抽搐、摇头等，也就是由"风"所引起的。又如冬天寒冷，可以引起水冻结冰，物体收缩的现象；那么在人体内，会引起血凝滞而运行不畅，出现抽筋的症状，也是由于"寒"所致。用自然现象来解释人体的生理或病理现象，这就解决了对人的生理或病理现象不可能采用直观方法来了解它的内部变化的难题。这在方法学上，是中医学很大的一个特点。

"天人相应"和"天人同理"的理论，都是根据人与自然界之间存在着统一性、人必然要受到自然界的制约的这一原理提出来的。它较正确地反映了人与自然的关系，是中医学理论的特点之一。

人的整体性原则是说人虽然是由脏腑、经络、形体、四肢、百骸、五官、九窍等所构成，但是一个整体。在人体和外界发生联系的时候，是以一个整体发生联系，而不是以各个部分发生联系的。《内经》认为人是一个"小天地"，是一个完整的系统。人体是以五脏为核心、以心为主导、以经络为道路而网络全身的有机的整体性结构。外界对人体发生作用虽然是在某个部位，但是它必然通过经络而作用到人体的核心部分，即由"心—五脏"构成的司令部而影响到全身。当人体对外界的作用发生反应的时候，也不是某一部位独自地作出反应，而是在"心—五脏"的指挥下作出反应。因此，人体任何一个部位发生的反应都是全身反应在局部的表现。人体任何一个部位的疾病，也是全身性疾病在局部的表现。根据这个原则，中医在处理疾病时，必须注意全身的情况，必须针对全身进行治疗。当然，重视整体，并不能忽视局部。正确处理好人体的整体和局部的关系，才能正确运用中医的整体性原则。

（3）确立了阴阳五行学说的指导地位　《内经》把以精气学说为基础的阴阳五行学说作为指导思想和方法论，贯穿于整个《内经》所建立起来的医学理论体系之中。并以阴阳平衡、阴阳的依存和制约以及五行承制的观点来认识人体的生理和病理过程，并指导临床辨证和治疗。

（4）创立了以五脏为核心，以心为主导的生理学结构——"藏象学说"　《内经》强调了人体的整体性原则，但对人体各组成部分不是平均地看待，而是突出了五脏的作用，创立了以五脏为核心、以心为主导、以经络为通路的生理学结构，组成在心神主宰下的五个生理系统（即心系统、肺系统、脾系统、肝系统、肾系统），以统率全身，构成一个有机的整体。以精、气、血、津液为生命物质，在心神的主宰下，五脏的协调下，经络的联系中进行有条不紊的生命活动。《灵枢·师传》说："五脏六腑，心为之主。"《素问·灵兰秘典论》说："凡此十二官者，不得相失也，故主明则下安，主不明则十二官危。"都是强调人体的整体性，强调了心的主宰作用。《内经》就是在这种生理结构观点的基础上，来认识人体的病理现象，并指导临床的辨证和治疗。这就是《内经》的"藏象学说"。

（5）创立了病因学和病机学理论　《内经》否定了神鬼惩罚的致病作用，提出了是由于人体和其周围环境之间或人体内部协调关系的破坏引起了疾病的发生，建立了以自然、社会、精神、生活等因素为主的病因学理论。并强调内因（人体正气，即人体的抗病机能）在发病中的重要意义。

《内经》以上述病因学观点来认识人体的病理过程，以人体内部协调关系的破坏来解释病理现象的出现，创立了以阴阳失调、邪正斗争、脏气不和、气血紊乱、经气不畅等为主的病机学理论。

（6）确立了诊断学和治疗学的基本原则　《内经》将阴阳五行学说、藏象学说等作为基本观点，以四诊和辨证为具体内容，按阴阳、脏腑、经脉、气血和病因来辨证疾病，用阴阳、四时、五脏、五色、五声、脉象等来辨认症状，建立了诊断学的基本原则。

《内经》在上述观点和方法的指导下，对于疾病的治疗提出了"未病先防""既病防变""不治已病治未病"的思想；早期诊断，早期治疗，"先安未受邪之地""治病必求其本"，正确处理标本关系；调理阴阳、调理脏气和经气、调和气血、扶正祛邪的基本治法；因时、因人、因地制宜等作为指导治疗的基本原则的治疗学思想。

（7）确立了养生学的基本原则　《内经》在"天人相应"和"六气"、情态等致病的理论指导下，提出了顺应自然、不违天时、虚怀无欲、避邪有时等养生防病的基本原则，也提出了节制饮食、注意劳作锻炼等作为防病、强身的基本方法。

《内经》的内容所涉及的范围甚广，从医学的基础理论到临床诊治的基本原则无所不包，从而确立了中医学理论的轮廓框架。直至今天，中医学理论虽然有很大的发展，但只是按照《内经》设计的中医学理论体系的框架进行充实和扩展，基本没有越出《内经》的理论体系。所以说《内经》的成书是中医学理论体系基本确立的标志。

《难经》又名《黄帝八十一难经》，是继《内经》之后又一本重要的医学理论著作。其成书时间已不可考，有说是在秦汉之际，有说是在东汉末年。相传为扁鹊所著，但不足为信。

《难经》全书分八十一难。论述了脉学、经络、脏腑、疾病的传变及预后、五腧穴、针刺手法等问题。其理论是本源于《内经》，但对《内经》的理论又有所发展。提出了"命门"一说，对三焦、元气的理论有重要的发挥。对后世医学理论的发展，产生了重大的影响。因为它对中医学理论体系的确立作出了重大的贡献，所以后世常把《内》《难》二书并称。

3. 《神农本草经》确立了中药学的理论体系

《内经》虽然对中药学和处方学提出了一些基本原则，但它毕竟不是药物和治疗方面的专著；而且《内经》是以针刺治疗为主的。因而，《内经》所提出的关于药物学和处方学的理论是不够的。

《神农本草经》（简称《本草经》）是现在可考的我国第一部中药学专著，其成书大约是在西汉平帝元始元年前后，其作者已不可考。原书早已散失，现行本是后世从历代本草书中集辑而成的，分为3卷。

《本草经》汇集了秦汉以前的中药学知识，以四气五味概括药物的性能，以寒热补泻来阐明药理作用，根据药物的有毒无毒及其作用，分为上、中、下三品。上品120味，功能益气，久服使人轻身成仙；中品120味，功能补虚，久服能强身壮体；下品125味，有毒，功能除邪，服之能祛邪治病。全书共载药物计

365 味。《本草经》还提出了君、臣、佐、使与七情合和的药物配伍和组方理论。《本草经》创立的药物学和处方学理论，为后世中药学和处方学理论确立了基本理论体系。所以说，《本草经》的成书，是中药学和处方学理论体系基本确立的标志。

《本草经》以上、中、下三品分类药物，临床实用价值不大，《素问·调经论》已提出不同的意见。其谓上品无毒，久服能轻身成仙，是反映秦汉时期寻求仙丹、以求长生不老的风气。中品之药，多为金石之品，不宜轻服。下品之药，其认为有毒，不可常用，其实正是祛邪治病之药，是临床常用的药物。

4.《伤寒杂病论》确立了中医临床医学理论体系

《内经》是医学理论专著，虽也涉及临床医学的问题，但对具体病种的诊断和治法失之于具体，难作临床医生之楷模。对于疾病的辨证，虽然《内经》也提出从病因、病位和邪正关系等方面进行辨证的原则，但是不够具体，后人难以效法。《神农本草经》是药物学专著，虽然提出了处方和药物配伍的基本原理，但怎样具体应用，问题并未解决。在这种情况下，《伤寒杂病论》作为一部临床医学专著，填补了这个空白。

《伤寒杂病论》共 16 卷，相传为东汉末年长沙太守张仲景所撰，大约成书于东汉献帝建安十五年（公元 210 年）。张氏撰用《素问》《九卷》（即《灵枢》的别名），《八十一难》《阴阳大论》《胎胪药录》和《平脉辨证》诸书，编成《伤寒杂病论》。他总结了汉以前的临床医学方面的成就，集当时医学之大成。书成后不久，因战乱而散佚，未能流传。至晋，经太医王叔和收集编纂成书，不久又散佚。到唐初孙思邈编《千金要方》

时，未能见到此书，只言"江南诸师秘仲景方不传"。至孙氏再编《千金翼方》时，才把《伤寒杂病论》的内容收集进去。至北宋·高保衡、林亿、孙奇等校正医书时，《伤寒杂病论》已被分为《伤寒论》和《金匮要略方论》二书。

《伤寒论》10卷22篇，立397法、113方，为外感热病之专著。本书创立了"六经辨证"的理法方药、辨证论治的临床医学理论体系，被后世推崇为"方书之祖"。《金匮要略方论》在北宋·高保衡等校正医书时早已亡佚。后来孙奇根据《金匮玉函要略方》一书，弃其第一卷"伤寒"部分，取其后二卷分为3卷，共25篇，262方，改名为《金匮方论》，即今所见之《金匮要略方论》。其为杂病之专著，创立了以"脏腑辨证"论杂病证治的临床医学理论体系，并提出"千般疢难，不越三条"的以"三因"分类病因的理论。宋·陈无择据此提出"三因说"。

《伤寒杂病论》的成书，为中医临床医学的理论体系定下了规范，使后人能够效仿。后世虽然在临床医学理论方面有很大的充实和发展，但仍然未越出《伤寒杂病论》所提出的理法方药的辨证论治体系。所以说，《伤寒杂病论》的成书是中医临床医学理论体系确立的标志。

中医学理论体系，从《内经》开始，到《伤寒杂病论》成书，即告完全确立。具体内容见图1。后世虽然对中医学理论也作出很大的贡献，并且有很大的发展，但在理论体系方面，只是起到充实和完善的作用，而没有根本性的改变。

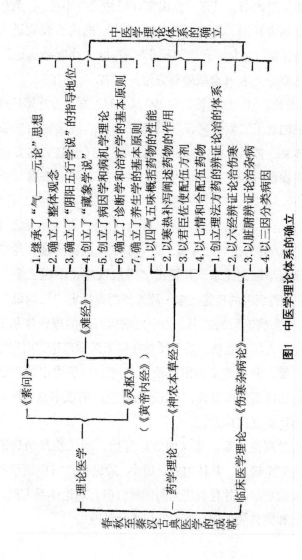

图1 中医学理论体系的确立

阴阳五行

阴阳五行是阴阳学说和五行学说的简称，是我国古典哲学中朴素的唯物论和自发的辩证法思想。阴阳学说和五行学说是古人从自然界及社会中概括出来的一般规律，并用以认识自然及社会现象，为先秦的主要哲学思想体系之一。

阴阳和五行的概念虽然早已形成，但直到战国末期，邹衍推演五行，把精气、阴阳和五行三种学说揉为一体，才形成阴阳五行学说，并成为一种盛行的哲学思想。正是这一时期，我国古代医学的发展进入了转折时刻，医学知识和医疗经验的积累已经相当丰富，开始向医学理论迈进，此时需要一种哲学思想作为指导，对大量的医学素材进行加工，使之系统化、理论化。在这种情况下，就把当时新兴的又极为盛行的阴阳五行学说引入医学中来，成为中医学理论的指导思想和方法论，在中医学中占据着特殊的地位。由于这样的原因，学习中医的人都必须学习并掌握阴阳五行学说。否则，就难以深入地研究并掌握中医学的理论体系。

阴阳五行学说毕竟是一种古代的哲学思想，深深地印着时代的烙印，本身存在着一定的缺陷。为此，我们在学习它的时候，必须以辩证唯物主义和历史唯物主义的观点和方法进行分析，取其精华，弃其糟粕，使它更好地为医学实践服务。

在中医学理论中，虽然主要是运用阴阳五行学说，但是为了学习的方便，有必要先予以分别介绍，而后再进行综合讨论。

一、阴阳学说

（一）阴阳的基本概念

1. 阴阳概念的形成

太阳一出来，一座山就有向着太阳的一面和背着太阳的一面，向着太阳的一面光亮而温暖，背着太阳的一面阴暗而湿冷。这不是某一座山所特有的，而只要是山，都存在着这种现象。远古的人们发现了这种现象，就把向着太阳一面的山坡称为"山之阳"或"阳坡"，把背着太阳的一面称为"山之阴"或"阴坡"，这就是最早对阴阳的应用。《山海经·南山经》说："又东三百七十里曰杻阳之山，其阳多赤金，其阴多白金。"意思是说：再向东去三百七十里，有座山叫杻阳山，在它的阳坡面多产赤金（指铜），在它的阴坡面多产白金（即锡）。《吕氏春秋·重己篇》说："室大则多阴，台高则多阳。"房室大了，太阳照不到的地方（阴）就多了；土也筑得高，得到太阳的照射（阳）就多了。这里所谈的"阴阳"都是太阳的照射而言。向着太阳，得到阳光照射的就称为"阳"；背着太阳，阳光照射不到的地方即称为"阴"。可见"阴阳"的最初涵义，仅是指对太阳的向背而言。"阴阳"的涵义是具体的、明确的，不是哲学上的抽象概念。

只要有山，就存在"山之阳"和"山之阴"的区别。山没有了，"山之阳"和"山之阴"也就不存在了。"山之阳"和"山之阴"是随山的存在而存在，随山的消失而消失。因此，古人就把它们看作是两种截然相反、但又存在于一山之中的山的

26

属性。

随着人们生活和劳动范围的扩大，知识积累的增加，逐渐认识到在一个事物的内部，存在着截然相反的两种属性，是有普遍性的。如宇宙就是由天和地构成的，天是轻清向上，是无形的；地是重浊向下，是有形的。一日是由白天和黑夜构成的，白天太阳升起，给人们带来了光明和温暖；黑夜太阳下山，月亮升起，给人以阴暗和寒冷。一日正是由于太阳和月亮所代表的两种截然不同的属性所构成的。一年四季的变化，出现了寒暑的交替，也正是由于寒暑的交替，给万物带来了生机和活力，引起了万物生长化收藏的变化。天气有晴雨的变化，给大地带来了欣欣向荣的景象。人有男女的不同，禽兽有雌雄的区别，正是这种性别上的差异，给人类和禽兽带来了性格、生活习惯等方面的差别，并保证了种族的繁衍，给人类社会和动物世界带来了繁荣昌盛。其他如山有高低，水有清浊，物有轻重，位置有上下、左右、前后、内外，方向有东西、南北，运动有动静、升降、快慢、进退，时间有迟早，物体有大小，战争有攻守、胜败，生命现象有幼老、生死等等，说明了两种截然相反的属性或现象，共存于一体之中而不能分离，构成一个相对独立的整体，是一种普遍的现象。世界上的万事万物正是由此而产生、而发展，并维持了世界的存在和延续。这种既相关联又相对立的两种属性，古人以"阴阳"来表示。这样，"阴阳"就从原来表示对阳光向背的具体概念，转变为不再具有具体内容的抽象概念，而成为哲学范畴。

"阴阳"是对自然界或社会中的事物或现象，既相关联又相对立的两类属性的概括。《灵枢·阴阳系日月》说："阴阳者，有名而无形。"即是说"阴阳"是有名称和涵义的，而没有具体形象和所指的，是抽象的概念。

"阴阳"作为一个抽象的概念，早在《内经》成书以前已经存在，并被用来说明医学中的某些问题。例如《左传》就记载医和以"六气"作为致病的原因，他说："六气曰阴、阳、风、雨、晦、明也。"他用"阴阳"表示"寒热"，并作为致病因素。但是，把"阴阳"作为一个抽象的哲学概念，在医学理论中广泛而全面地应用，成为中医学理论体系中的重要组成部分，则是从《内经》开始的。

《内经》在继承前人对"阴阳"理解的基础上，将它引入医学理论，用来认识和解释医学中的理论问题。《素问·阴阳应象大论》说："阴阳者，天地之道也，万物之纲纪，变化之父母，生杀之本始，神明之府也，治病必求其本。""阴阳"是自然界最根本的规律，万物都可以用"阴阳"来进行分类，使之提纲挈领，进行概括。世界上万物发生变化，是产生于"阴阳"；一个生命的产生和消亡，是由"阴阳"引起的；生命现象的表现，它的根源是存在于"阴阳"之中；所以疾病也是由"阴阳"引起的，治病就必须寻求"阴阳"这个根本所在。《内经》继承了前人把"阴阳"当作世界运动变化的根本规律的观点，引申出"阴阳"也是医学中的根本规律。《素问·宝命全形论》说："人生有形，不离阴阳。"人的生命所表现出来的各种现象，都离不开"阴阳"这个根本原因。《灵枢·病传》说："明于阴阳，如惑之解，如醉之醒。"只要明了了"阴阳"的道理，就好像遇到了迷惑不解的问题，马上就能得到解决一样；又好像一个饮醉了酒的人，马上就能使他酒醒脑清。《内经》把阴阳学说当作方法论来看，它能使人的思路开阔，聪敏智慧，是解决问题最有效的方法。

《内经》把阴阳学说运用到医学的各个方面，包括对人体的解剖、生理、病因、发病、病机以及临床医学的诊断、辨证、治疗和预防等各个方面，都运用阴阳学说的理论和法则来进行分析和认识，以致把阴阳学说作为中医学理论体系的指导思想和方法论，而占有特殊的位置。

2. 阴阳的整体性

"阴阳"是对自然界或社会中的事物或现象既相关联又相对立的两类属性的概括，说明"阴阳"之间既存在着对立性，又存在着统一性。两个相互对立的属性之间，如没有统一性，就不存在"阴阳"的关系。所以，"阴阳"的双方只能存在于一个相对独立的整体之中。只有当两个事物或现象之间发生了具体的联系，构成为一个相对独立的整体时，才能构成"阴阳"的关系。

在进行理论分析时，男和女就是一对"阴阳"关系。因为男性和女性都是人，共同构成了人类社会，这就是他们之间的统一性；而男性和女性由于性别上的差异，在性情、心理和习惯上的不同，在社会分工中的不同，这就是他们之间的对立性。正因为这样的原因，男性和女性构成了一对"阴阳"关系。但这并不是说，任何一个男性和任何一个女性都是"阴阳"关系。如果某一男性和另一女性，生死不相往来，从未发生过任何的联系，那就不构成"阴阳"关系。在具体生活中，不仅男女之间可以构成"阴阳"关系，而且在男性之间或女性之间都可以构成"阴阳"关系，只要在两人之间发生了某种方式的联系。比如共同完成某一项工作，或对某一问题两人持不同的意见，或两人参加了同一项目的竞赛等，只要将两人联系在一起，构成了一个相对独立的整体，就构成了"阴阳"的关系。当这样联系一旦中断，这个相对独立的整体不再存在，已构成的"阴阳"关系也随之消失。再如，在一般情况下，物体的硬度和运动的速度是两个不同范畴的概念，二者互不相关。因而就不能构成"阴阳"的关系。但是，二者均和物体的温度有关，物体在进行高速运动的时刻，必然要引起它温度的变化，温度的改变又可以引起物体的硬度变化。因此，研究物体在高速运动时的硬度变化，由于温度把二者联系在一起，其速度和硬度也就构成了一对"阴阳"关系。

所以，事物或现象之间是否存在着"阴阳"关系，取决于它们之间是否存在着对立统一的关系，是否发生了具体的联系，能否构成一个相对独立的整体，"阴阳"的关系只存在于发生了具体联系的事物或现象之间，只存在于一个相对独立的整体之中。不发生具体联系，不存在于一个相对独立的整体之中的事物或现象，是不存在着"阴阳"关系，这就是"阴阳"的整体性。

3. 阴阳的相对性和属性的规定性

（1）阴阳的相对性　"阴阳"的相对性，一是说"阴阳"本身就是一种相对的概念。"阴阳"的涵义最初就是对阳光的向背而言，这就是相对的概念。一座高山，一面向着太阳，另一面就背着太阳。如果没有向着太阳的一面，背着太阳的一面也就不存在了。这两面共存于一山之中，是不能分离的，是在比较中存在的。"阴阳"还被用来表示温度的高低、冷热，运动的快慢、动静，物体的轻重，反应的敏捷和迟钝等。这些都是相对的概念，都是在比较中存在的。例如我们坐在电视机旁观看国家女子排球队的比赛时，虽然队员们的身高多数是在 1.8 米以上，但是，却没有给我们留下身材高大的印象，因为队员们的身材都高。如果一个身材不高的工作人员走近她们的身旁，这时才察觉到，这些女将的身材是高大的。因为这时有了对比，因此才显出了她们的高大。"人到黄山不爬山"，一是说黄山风景之美，无以相比；二是说黄山之高，耸入云霄之中。登于黄山之巅，立于云雾之中，如临仙境，确属胜观。如果我们考虑一下黄山的海拔高度，黄山中最高的莲花峰也只有1873米高，和青海高原比较还低一千多米，和西藏高原比较，还不足它的一半高，更无法和高原上的高山比高低了。就是高原上的一个洼地，也要比黄山高出几百米或千米。黄山是在低海拔当中破土而出，周围没有能和它相比的，所以就显得它特别高。高原中的洼地，处于环山包围之中，更显出它的低洼，而实际上它却比黄山高。所以，高低、上下、冷热、快慢、胖瘦等只有在对比中才能显示出来。高和低比、上与下比、冷和热比、快与慢比、胖和瘦比，没有比较，这些概念就难以建立。对比的条件发生了变化，给人的印象也就随即改变。所以，用"阴阳"来表示的双方，它们只存在于相比之中，只是一种相对的概念，而不是绝对的概念。

"阴阳"的相对性，第二种意思是说，"阴阳"是一种抽象的概念，而不是指具体的事物或现象。在讨论具体问题时，"阴阳"所表示的具体内容，是随着讨论的问题而确定的。如我们所讨论的问题是物体的位置，"阴阳"所表示的内容可能是指上下、高低、前后、左右或内外；讨论的问题是物体在具体环境中的运动，"阴阳"就可能是表示快慢、出入、升降或动静；如讨论的问题是疾病的发生，"阴阳"可能是表示邪正、气血、营卫等。所以，"阴阳"所表示的具体内容是随着讨论问题的内容而决定的，"阴阳"本身不表示任何固定不变的内容或具体的事物或现象。

中医书中常用"阴阳"来表示一定的内容，在不同的地方，"阴阳"的涵义是不同的。《素问·金匮真言论》说："夫言人之阴阳，则外为阳，内为阴；言人身之阴阳，则背为阳，腹为阴；言人身之脏腑中阴阳，则脏者为阴，腑者为阳。"在这段话中，"阴阳"的涵义各不相同。第一是从整体的内外而言，所以说体表为阳、体内为阴；第二是从人身的体表而言，所以说背面为阳，腹面为阴；第三是从内脏而言，根据脏和腑的特性，所以说五脏为阴，六腑为阳。这三句话是因为讨论问题的范围发生变化，所以"阴阳"的含义也随之改变。《素问·阴阳应象大论》说："暴怒伤阴，暴喜伤阳。"这里的"阴"是指"阴脏"，即指肝；"阳"是"阳脏"，即心，和前面的"阴阳"涵义又不相同。《素问·调经论》说："夫邪之生也，或生于阴，或生于阳。其生于阳者，得之风雨寒暑；其生于阴者，得之饮食居处，阴阳喜怒。"这一段话中三对"阴阳"的涵义也不相同。前两对"阴阳"是讲发病的部位，"生于阴"是说病发于内，是指脏腑；"生于阳"是说病发于表，即指肌肤。最后的一个"阴阳"是讲致病因素，它所指的是男女房室之劳。中医书中对阴阳的运用是很广泛的，必须根据整句话或整段文字的意思来判断。

"阴阳"的相对性，还表示为对一个具体事物或现象的"阴阳"属性的判断。比如我们讨论温度的范围是限制在0℃～10℃之间，那么0℃为阴，10℃属"阳"；如温度范围变为10℃～100℃之间，则10℃为"阴"，100℃为"阳"。10℃既可以属"阴"，也可以属"阳"，这是取决于讨论问题的前题。前题变了，具体事物或现象的"阴阳"属性也随之而变。这就是说，具体事物的"阴阳"属性不是固定的，是相对的，是随着对比的标准而发生变化。所以在《素问·金匮真言论》里，把五脏归于"阴"，腑归于"阳"；而在五脏之中，又根据所在的位置，把心肺归之于"阳"，把脾肝肾归之于"阴"；在心肺之中，又把心作为"阳中之阳"，肺为"阳中之阴"；在脾肝肾当中，把肝作为"阴中之阳"，肾为"阴中之阴"，脾为"阴中之至阴"。这些都是根据对比的关系，来说明五脏的"阴阳"属性。

（2）阴阳属性的规定性　"阴阳"是相对的概念，它不是指某一具体的事物或现象，是根据讨论的问题而确定它的所指。但是，"阴阳"的属性是有规定性的，在讨论问题的范围被确定以后，在这问题中所包含的双方，谁属于"阴"，谁属于"阳"，是确定的，不能更换的。比如在研究物体的温度时，温度高的为"阳"，温度低的为"阴"；温度上升的为"阳"，温度下降的为"阴"。在研究物体的运动状态时，主要运动的为"阳"，被动运动的为"阴"；处于运动状态的为"阳"，处于静止状态的为"阴"；运动快的为"阳"，运动慢的为"阴"；作上升运动的为"阳"，作下降运动的为"阴"；处于加速运动的为"阳"，处于减速运动的属"阴"。在研究动能状态时，功能亢进的为"阳"，功能衰退的为"阴"；处于兴奋状态的为"阳"，处于抑制状态的为"阴"；功能在逐渐加强的为"阳"，功能在逐步减退的为"阴"。在研究动物的性别上，雄性的为"阳"，雌性的为"阴"；比较凶猛的雌性动物为"阴中之阳"，比较温柔的雄性动物为"阳中之阴"。在这些问题上，"阴阳"的双方是不能对换的。

"阴阳"的属性具有规定性，这是因为"阴阳"的最初涵义是指具体的现象，即对阳光的向背。虽然后来"阴阳"被抽象化了，但是，"阴阳"的涵义并没有完全脱离它原始的涵义。阳光给自然界带来了光明、温暖、生气和欣欣向荣；离开了阳光就意味着黑暗、寒冷、死亡和万物沉寂。因而概括出：凡是光亮的、温暖的、上升的、活跃的、好动的、主动的、外向性的、功能性的、亢进的、无形的、清晰的、生长的、增加的、富有竞争性的等都属于"阳"的特性；与此相反，凡属于黑暗的、寒冷的、下降的、沉静的、被动的、内向性的、物质性的、衰退的、有形的、混浊的、枯萎的、减少的、富有妥协性的等都属于"阴"的特性。"阴阳"的特性都是从它原始的涵义中引伸出来的。对具体事物或现象的属性进行分析时，就要根据"阴阳"的属性与具体事物或现象的属性进行类比，从而作出判断，归属于"阴阳"两类之中。如在研究液体的透明度时，清彻透明、清稀的液体更接近于无形，给人以明亮的感觉，所以属"阳"；混浊不清、黏稠的液体更接近于有形，给人以阴暗的感觉，所以属"阴"。在研究性别时，不论是人或动物，雌性的性格趋向于内向性、好静、温柔、偏于妥协，所以属"阴"；雄性的性格趋向于外向性、好动、暴躁、偏于好斗，所以属阳。

由于"阴阳"的属性具有规定性，所以，在讨论的问题被确定以后，问题的双方，属"阴"属"阳"就要根据"阴阳"的特性来进行判断，是不能随便乱配的。

（3）矛盾和阴阳的关系　矛盾是对立统一的概念，也是相对的概念，而不是专指某一具体的事物或现象，它的具体涵义也要根据所讨论的问题来确定。在这些方面，"矛盾"和"阴阳"

是相同的。但是，"矛盾"的属性是没有规定性的，"矛盾"的双方是可以互换的。以上下为例，既可把上作为"矛"，把下作为"盾"，也可把下作为"矛"，上作为"盾"，都不影响问题的讨论。而在"阴阳"中，上只能作为"阳"，下只能作为"阴"，二者是不能互换的。在这一点上，"矛盾"和"阴阳"是不同的，阴阳的相对性是有条件的，是不彻底的；而"矛盾"的相对性是无条件的，是彻底的。因此，在应用时，"阴阳"的应用是有条件的，有限制的；而"矛盾"的应用是无条件的，没有限制的。由于这样的原因，用"矛盾"来代替"阴阳"是不行的，二者的概念是有区别的。

4. 阴阳的可分性

"阴阳"是可分的，即"阴阳"之中还可分"阴阳"，并可以一直分下去，其中仍包含"阴阳"双方。《素问·阴阳离合论》说："阴阳者，数之可十，推之可百；数之可千，推之可万。万之大，不可胜数，然其要一也。"就是说"阴阳"可以无穷尽地分下去，分至千万，但它最根本的方法只有一个，即"阴阳"的方法。

"阴阳"是可分的，一直分到最小的程度，仍包含"阴阳"两部分。例如一块磁铁，它包含 N 和 S 两极。磁铁可按"一分为二"的方法分下去，一直分到最小的程度，只要它还有磁铁性，它就必然仍包含 N 和 S 两极。

一个物体具可分性，被分成的每一部分仍具有相对的完整性，这说明了物体结构的层次性。例如全息照像，照片中的任何一点，一经放大，又是一张完整的照片。又如人体的结构，是以五脏为中心的五个生理系统结合组成的。每个生理系统又是一个相对独立的整体，是由脏、腑、体、窍等所构成的。而这些脏、腑、体、窍又都有自己的相对独立性。各脏腑又有自己的气血、津液、阴阳等物质。人体就是这样由不同的层次所构成的，各生理系统相互配合、相互协调，组成了一个严密的、有机的整体，维持了人的生命功能。

（二）阴阳学说的基本内容

1. 阴阳学说的基本观点

阴阳学说认为世界是由"阴阳"二气所构成的，"阴阳"二气是处于不断的运动之中；由于"阴阳"的运动，引起了世界万物的发生、发展和变化；又由于"阴阳"运动形式的不同，产生了世界万物的差异性；"阴阳"二气相互依存、互为根源，而又相互对立、相互制约，它引起了"阴阳"的消长变化和相互转化。在方法上，阴阳学说就是"一分为二"的方法。这些内容将在有关的部分介绍，这里只讨论如下两个问题：

（1）"平衡论"的观点　阴阳学说是古人从生活、自然及社会现象中概括出来的一般规律性。在远古时期，社会生产力极为低下，人类的生活是衣不能暖身、食不能饱腹，每天为"吃住"问题而奔波。在这样的生活条件下，衣暖食饱是当时人们的最大愿望，把自给自足当作理想社会来描述，而不敢有更大的要求。阴阳学说正是产生在这样经济基础之上的社会环境之中，这是产生"平衡论"的社会根源。

阴阳学说是在春秋战国时期逐步完善的。春秋战国时期正是群雄争霸之际。在这样的条件下，一个弱小国家要求得生存，就必然要搞力量平衡。弱小者跻身于群雄之间，就要附翼于强国之下，并在七雄之间制造相互牵制的因素，以便在剩余的缝隙间求生。阴阳学说是在这一时期完善的，不可能不受到当时"平衡论"和"牵制论"的影响。所以，在阴阳学说中处理"阴阳"之间的关系时，就采用了"平衡"和"牵制"这两种方法。

在自然界，"平衡"也是维护事物稳定的一种基本方式，生态平衡就是例子。肥料——植物——食草动物——食肉动物组成了一条生物链，它们之间的平衡，是维持他们之间同步发展的必要条件。动物的尸体和粪便为植物生长提供了肥料，植物又成为食草动物的饲料，食草动物又为食肉动物提供了食物，它们之间只有处于平衡状态，才能同步地发展。其中任何一个环节发生变化，都要引起其他环节的同步反应。如发生了旱灾，植物的减产，就要引起食草动物的饥饿和死亡。食肉动物也要伴随食草动物的减少而发生食物不足，引起相应的减少。大自然正是通过这种方式来调节或控制生物的发展，使它们不能无限制地繁殖和增加，以维持生态平衡。

在人类社会中，性别之间也必须处于平衡状态。这种平衡一旦被打破，就要成为社会的不安定因素。所幸的是，在大自然的控制之下，男女的数量只是小范围内波动，在总体上是平衡的。这对社会的安定、人类的进步是有重要的意义。

用人工来控制子女的性别，必将导致性别平衡的打破，带来严重的社会问题，是不可取的方法。

《内经》用阴阳学说来阐述医学理论问题，是持"平衡论"的观点。《素问·生气通天论》说："阴平阳秘，精神乃治。"阴阳平衡，方能秘藏而不外泄，人的精神就能保持正常。《素问·调经论》说："夫阴与阳皆有俞会，阳注于阴，阴满于外，阴阳匀平，以充其形，九候若一，命曰平人。"阴经和阳经在俞穴交会，气血在阳经充盈后就注入阴经，在阴经中充满后又外溢于阳经。这样阴经和阳经内的气血都均匀而平衡，以此来充养人身。人身得到气血均匀的充养，各部的功能正常，所以三部九候的脉象都是一样的，没有偏盛偏衰的现象，这样的人就称为"平人"，即正常的人。《素问·至真要大论》说："谨察阴阳所在而调之，以平为期。"仔细地察看阴阳偏盛偏衰发生的部位而进行调治，以恢复它的平衡为限度。《内经》认为阴阳平衡是人体生理状态的表现，而阴阳平衡的破坏是病理状态的表现。所以，医生治病的关键就在于调理阴阳，恢复阴阳的平衡，人体也就恢复了正常。

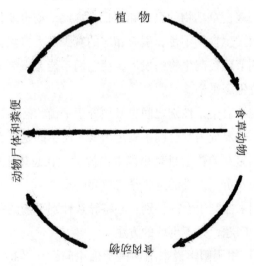

图2 植物和动物间的生态平衡图

说明：植物减少，食草动物缺乏饲料而减少，食肉动物也因食物缺乏而减少。大量动物因饥饿而死亡，动物尸体使土地肥料增加，为下一年度的植物增产准备了条件。植物增产又促进了食草、食肉动物的增加。但由于土地面积的限制，植物增产被限制，动物也不能无限制地增加，而只能处于植物和动物之间的平衡状态。

《内经》强调阴阳平衡的观点和医学研究的范围有关。医学的目的是保护人体的健康和延长人的寿命，医学研究的范围是局限在正常人和病人之间，促使病人恢复正常。阴阳平衡是人体健康的必要条件，所以要维护人体的健康和长寿，就必须维护阴阳平衡。由于这样的原因，《内经》就坚持了"平衡论"的观点。

（2）以阳气为主导的观点　阴阳学说是建立在"平衡论"的基础之上的，这并不意味阴阳占有同等的位置。《内经》的观点是以阳气为主导。《素问·生气通天论》说："阳气者，若天与日。失其所，则折寿而不彰。故天运当以日光明。"人体中的阳气，就好象天体和太阳的关系一样。天体本身并不发光，也不能给大自然以生机。大自然的光明和生机，是太阳给予的。太阳给大自然以光明、温暖，万物才有了生机，才有盛衰的变化。如果太阳失去了它应有的地位，不能发挥它的作用，自然界的生命现象就要夭折，万物的盛衰变化就不能再显示出来。所以，天体的运转应当让太阳充分发挥它给自然界以光明和温暖的作用。《内经》强调了阳光在自然界中的重要性，是产生生命现象的根本原因。同样地，在人体的生命过程中，阳气也是占主导地位。

《内经》为什么以阳气为主导？可以从以下几方面来理解。

一是从古人对生命起源的认识来看。《河图·序》说："天一生水，地六成之；地二生火，天七成之；天三生木，地八成之；地四生金，天九成之；天五生土，地十成之。"这里面包含有几个观点：一是任何新生命的产生，都有发生和成熟这两个过程。所以，五行的生成都有"生"和"成"这两个数，表示发生和成熟这两个过程。第二是任何一个新生命的产生都是由阴精和阳气交感而成，阳生于阴而成于阳，阴生于阳而成于阴，"生数"和"成数"就包含了阴阳交感和阴阳互根的原理。第三是说在生命的起源过程中，首先是生成水，这为生命的起源准备了条件。但是，只有水还不能产生生命，还必须有火，只有在一定温度的条件下，即水火相交，才能产生生命。生命起源于水中，而后才出现各种生命。水是产生生命的必要条件，但是，只有在火的作用下，水火相交，生命才能产生。所以，火（阳气）是一个关键性因素。

二是从自然界的生命现象来看，阳光给生物带来了生机。没有阳光，就没有光明和温暖，多数植物的萌芽、生长、开花、结果就不可能发生，动物的生命也受到威胁。阳光给自然界带来了欣欣向荣的景象。在热带和亚热带地区，植物生长茂盛，动物繁殖旺盛；而寒带地区，则植物生长迟缓，甚至不能生长，动物也寥寥无几。这些现象都说明了阳光、温度对生命的重要性，也就说明了阳气对生命的重要性。

三是从生命现象来看。活人和死人在形态结构上并无不同，但二者又有本质的区别，活人有生命现象，死人则无。在古代的条件下，最易被发现的是死人没有呼吸，体温降低，这是没有阳气的表现。活人有阳气的温煦，所以能呼吸，体温正常，并带动了一切生理功能；死人没有阳气，呼吸停止，体温丧失，一切生理功能也因而停止。从这个角度来说，人的生死，是取决于阳气的有无，而不是取决于形体。这说明了阳气对生命的重要意义，在人体生命中占主导地位。当然，阳气只有附着于形体之上，才能有生命现象，对生命才有意义。没有形体的存在，阳气对生命也就失去了意义。

四是从死亡过程来看。人的死亡虽然可以由各种原因引起，但其最终没有阳气的亡越，就不至于死亡。阳气亡越是死亡的直接原因，亡阴、失血、脱汗，只有导致阳气亡越，这才引起了死亡。

以上都说明阳气对生命的重要意义，所以《内经》是以阳气为主导，并以这种观点来解释人体的生理与病理现象。强调阳气的主导作用，并不否定阴气的重要性。《类经图翼》说："阴无阳不生，阳无阴不成。"古人提出的"孤阴不生，独阳不长"，都说明"阴阳"的依存和互根，"阴阳"是共存于一体之中，不能分离。《素问·生气通天论》说："凡阴阳之要，阳密乃固。两者不和，若春无秋，若冬无夏。因而和之，是谓圣度。故阳强不能密，阴气乃绝；阴平阳秘，精神乃治；阴阳离决，精气乃绝。"这段论述，强调了阳气起主导作用，又说明了阴阳平衡和阴阳依存、互根的重要性，阴阳的分离，就导致了死亡。

2. 阴阳分类法

阴阳学说，实质上是一种分类法。《类经·阴阳类》说："阴阳者，一分为二也。"张景岳认为，阴阳就是两分法。

《内经》首先提出了"阴阳应象"的命题。"应"是相应、相合的意思，"象"是指事物或现象的外在表象或征象。"阴阳应象"即是说，自然界的事物或现象都有一定的表象或征象，这种表象或征象是和阴阳相应的。根据这种相应的关系，就可以把自然界的事物或现象归属于阴阳这两类之中，这就是阴阳分类法。

阴阳分类法是以阴阳的属性为依据，把事物或现象的外在表

41

现，和阴阳属性进行类比，归属于阴阳之中。《素问·阴阳应象大论》说："故积阳为天，积阴为地；阴静阳躁；阳生阴长，阳杀阴藏；阳化气、阴成形……水为阴、火为阳……阴味出下窍，阳气出上窍；味厚者为阴，薄为阴之阳；气厚者为阳，薄为阳之阴。"这都是以阴阳的属性为依据，和某些现象进行类比，从而归属于阴阳两类之中。并以阴阳的属性，来说明这些现象发生的机理。

相互关联又相互对立的现象是普遍存在的，所以，阴阳分类法具有广泛的意义。如数学中的加和减、乘和除，力学中的作用力和反作用力，化学中的化合与分解等，都可以分别归属于阴阳两类之中。具体见下表。

阴阳分类举例表

属　性	自然现象	空间位置	运动状态	生命现象	
阳	天日昼晴	外上前右	动升浮进	生长	发育
阴	地月夜雨	内下后左	静降沉退	衰老	成熟

属性	时间	形　质		温度		亮度	功能状态		厚度	透明	速度	重量
阳	早	无形	功能	温	热	明	兴奋	亢进	薄	清	快	轻
阴	迟	有形	物质	凉	寒	暗	抑制	衰退	厚	浊	慢	重

属性	力学	物质状态		电学	化学	引力	密度	
阳	作用力	气态	液态	正电	分解	排斥力	稀	疏
阴	反作用力	液态	固态	负电	化合	吸引力	稠	密

阴阳分类法也用于人体，如体表为阳，体内为阴；上半身为

42

阳，下半身为阴；背面为阳，腹面为阴；四肢为阳，躯干为阴；六腑为阳，五脏为阴；气为阳，血为阴；津为阳，液为阴；上窍（眼、耳、口、鼻）为阳，下窍（二阴）为阴等。还可把人体的生理、病理现象也归属于阴阳两类之中。

阴阳分类法的意义主要有两点：一是把自然界的事物或现象归属于阴阳两类之中，这就可以用阴阳学说的原理对自然界的事物或现象进行解释。其中也包括对人体的结构、生理或病理现象进行解释。二是通过阴阳分类法把自然界和人体联系起来，"天人一体""天人相应"的理论具体化，为中医的病因和病机学说的理论提供了依据。

天人的阴阳相互感应的思想，是中医学理论的基本观点之一，它贯穿于中医学理论的各个部分，中医学的藏象学说、经络学说、病因学说、病机学说以及临床医学中的诊断、治疗和预防的理论，无不建立在这种思想的基础之上。而天人的阴阳相互感应的思想，正是建立在阴阳分类法的基础之上。

3. 阴阳的联系方式

《内经》提出了"阴阳离合"的命题，正是对阴阳联系方式的概括。

"离"就是分离、排斥的意思；"合"就是结合、吸引的意思。"阴阳离合"是说阴阳之间能分能合，既相互排斥而又相互吸引，是对立统一的关系。阴阳能分能合，分之为二，合则为一，是分中有合，合中有分。

《灵枢·阴阳系日月》说："夫阴阳者，有名而无形，故数之可十，离之可百，散之可千，推之可万，此之谓也。"这就说明阴阳有离散特性的一方面，即阴阳的可分性。阴阳除按"一

43

分为二"的方式离散外，还可以按"一分为三"的方式离散，即成"三阴三阳"。"三阳"之离，则为太阳、阳明、少阳；"三阳"之合，则为"一阳"。"三阴"之离，则为太阴、厥阴、少阴；"三阴"之合，则为"一阴"。"一阴阳"离则为"三阴三阳"，"三阴三阳"合则为"一阴阳"。"三阴三阳"合而为"一"，即成为一个整体。实际上，"阴阳离合"就是讲阴阳的对立与统一，即互制与互生的关系。

在阴阳的"离合"中，是以"合"为主。因为没有"合"，没有阴阳之间的统一性，就不能构成"阴阳"的关系。只有二者之间存在着统一性，共存于一体之中，才能构成"阴阳"的关系。《素问·阴阳离合论》说："阳予之正，阴为之主。"就是强调"阴阳"之间的协调和统一，即"阴阳"只能存在于一体之中。但是，阴阳的"离"也是重要的。阴阳的相"离"，就是"阴阳"之间的对立与制约。没有阴阳的相"离"，就不可能有阴阳的相"合"。正是由于阴阳的"离合"，引起了阴阳的运动，导致了事物变化。

（1）阴阳的依存和互根　物质世界本身就是由阴阳二气所构成的，由于阴阳二气相互搏结，产生了具体的物质。又由于阴阳运动表现为不同的形式，这就引起了物质间的差异，产生了万物。所以，在具体的事物或现象中，必然存在着阴阳这两个组成部分。

阴阳，都是以对方的存在为其自身存在的先决条件。如上和下、高和低，都是在对比中得出来的概念，上是在和下进行对比，才知它是在上；高只有和低进行对比，才显出它高，没有下的存在，上就不能存在；没有低和高对比，高就显示不出来。其

44

他如升和降、浮和沉、动和静、雄和雌、男和女、胖和瘦、易和难、快和慢等，都是相对的概念，都是在对比中存在的。如果它的对立面不存在，其本身也就不能存在。

《素问·阴阳应象大论》说："阴在内，阳之守也；阳在外，阴之使也。"阴气在内，收敛阳气，使在外面表现出来的阳气，不至于耗散；表现在外面的阳气，是内部阴气的表现。这就强调了阴阳之间的依存关系，二者只能共存于一体之中。如从人体而言，则阴是指物质性的脏腑，阳则是脏腑功能在外面的表现。脏腑处于体内，它是显示于外的生命功能的依附；显示在外的生命的功能，是体内脏腑的功能表现。体内脏腑正常，与其相应的功能表现就正常。体内脏腑不正常，与其相应的功能表现就不正常。体外生命功能只能随体内脏腑的状态而表现，所以说"阴在内，阳之守也"。体外生命功能是体内脏腑的表现，所以说"阳在外，阴之使也"。无功能的脏腑是不成其为脏腑，无脏腑的功能是无本之木，是不存在的。所以，阴阳双方都是以对方的存在为其自身存在的先决条件；若对方不存在，则其自身就失去了存在的条件。这就是阴阳之间的依存性。

阴阳双方都要依赖对方才能生长变化，即阴的生长变化要依赖于阳的作用，阳的生长变化同样依赖于阴的作用。这里包括两层意思：一是说阴阳均要依赖对方，才能发挥作用；二是说阴阳可以相互转化。

例如，机床要发挥作用，必须要有动力。没有动力，机床只是一堆废铁。机床加上了动力，就能生产出产品，成为有用的工具。机床和产品均有形，属阴；动力无形属阳。说明了阴的生长变化要依赖于阳。电力是常用的动力，不管是水力发电或火力发电，但都必须带动发电机转动，才能发出电。说明了电的产生，必须依赖发电机，即阳的生长变化，要依赖于阴。

阴阳可以相互转化，阴可以转化为阳，阳可以转化为阴。如皮球在弹跳过程中，随着皮球弹跳的升高，动能逐渐减小，势能逐渐增加；随着皮球的下落，位置的降低，势能逐渐减小，动能逐渐增加。势能是随物体位置的抬高而增加，动能是随物体下降的加速度而增加。势能属阴，动能属阳。势能和动能之间的转化，就是阴阳转化的例子。

阴阳均赖对方而发挥作用和阴阳间的相互转化，都是阴阳间的互生、互根和互用作用，即阴能生阳，阳能生阴。在实际情况下，这两种方式共同发挥作用。在人体的生长发育过程中，要不断地从外界摄取营养的物质，转化为人体的组成部分，使身体成长，脏腑组织发育完善。同时也促使人体生命功能的增强和完善。这个过程是相当复杂的，阴阳的相互作用，促使对方的增长和完善；阴阳的相互转化，使双方共同达到更高的水平。《类经图翼》说："阴无阳不生，阳无阴不成。"就是强调阴阳间的互生、互根、互用的作用，这就是阴阳间的互根性。

阴阳之间的依存性和互根性，把阴阳双方联为一体，这就是阴阳的统一性。没有阴阳的统一性，二者不共存于一体之中，就不能构成阴阳的关系，也就谈不上阴阳的对立和制约。

（2）阴阳的对立和制约　阴阳的对立和制约是阴阳之间的第二种关系，但是，它是维持阴阳平衡的关键因素，是维持事物稳定状态的必备要素。

一个事物要存在下去，其内部必须处于稳定的状态。事物内部状态的稳定程度，决定了该事物的存在能力。以元素的化学活性为例，元素的化学活性取决于它原子的结构。原子是由中心部位带正电荷的原子核和围绕原子核在不同壳层上旋转的带负电荷的电子所构成。原子结构的稳定性取决于两个条件：一是原子核所带的正电荷数值要和在原子核外旋转的电子数相等；二是在不同能级壳层上的电子数要满足一定的量。满足了以上两个条件，它既不易丢失电子，也不能获得电子，这种原子结构具有很大的稳定性，常见的惰性元素的原子结构，就满足了上述的要求。多数元素的原子结构只能满足于第一个条件，即只能满足电荷间的平衡，没有满足力的平衡。所以，都是处于有条件的稳定状态，都具有化学活性，或是易于丢失电子，或是易于获得电子，获得电子或丢失了电子，打破了电荷间的平衡，转化为离子状态，就失去了它的稳定性。

失去或获得电子的原子转化为离子，由于原有的电荷平衡已被破坏，因而具有活泼的化学性质。离子不能单独存在，它必须和带有相反电荷而数值相等的离子结合，从而又满足了电荷之间的平衡以及力的平衡，恢复了物质的稳定性。和原子的结构不同的是，其最外层的电子是两个或两个以上不同的原子核所共用的。两个或两个以上不同离子结合在一起，就形成了化合物的分子，又恢复了它的稳定状态。

以人体而言，要保持人体的健康状态，就必须使人体的生命功能稳定在正常范围之内，即体内阴阳双方必须维持在正常的平衡状态之中。阴阳平衡的破坏，就意味着生命功能的失常，即为疾病现象。所以《素问·生气通天论》说："阴平阳秘，精神乃治；阴阳离决，精气乃绝。"

以上事实说明，阴阳平衡是自然界的事物或现象维持其稳定状态的常见方式和必要条件。阴阳平衡遭到破坏，事物或现象的稳定状态也随之丧失。

阴阳的平衡是一种什么样的平衡呢？概括的说，阴阳平衡是一种相对的平衡、动态的平衡、恒量的平衡，而且还是一种功能态的平衡。

阴阳是一种相对的平衡，即是说在阴阳之间，允许有一定范围的不平衡，只要这种不平衡不足以危及事物的稳定性，它就是属于阴阳平衡的范围。具体见图3。

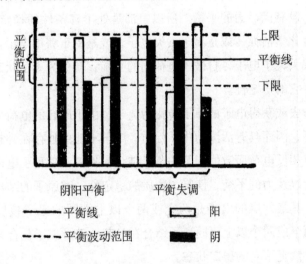

图3 阴阳的相对平衡图

说明：在坐标图中，在平衡范围内，实线只是理论上的平衡数值，虚线是表示平衡允许的波动范围。阴阳双方只要在虚线的范围内，既使在数值上并不平衡，由于它不危及事物的稳定性，仍属于平衡。只要阴阳双方有一方高于或低于平衡允许的波动范围，即为平衡失调。

48

从物质的三种状态来看，在一般情况下，水在 0 ℃ 以下为固态。0 ℃ ~ 100 ℃ 间为液态，100 ℃ 以上为气态。因此，当温度在 0 ℃ ~ 100 ℃ 之间波动，水的液态相当稳定。只有温度超过 100 ℃ 或低于 0 ℃ 时，水的液态才被破坏。有的物质的液态所允许的范围很小，其液化温度几乎就是它的气化温度，所以它的液态很不稳定。

人的生命也只能在一定的环境中正常的活动，超出了这个范围，人的生命就要受到威胁。如人体细胞外液的 pH 值为 7.35 ~ 7.45，在这范围内波动，对人的生命功能没有影响。如果 pH 值的波动范围超过了上述范围，就要引起酸中毒或碱中毒，人的正常生命活动就不能维持。

以上例子说明，阴阳平衡经常有一个允许的波动范围。在波动范围内波动，即使阴阳不平衡，也不会危及事物的稳定性，所以仍把它当作是平衡的，这就是相对平衡的涵义。

相对平衡的意义在于它扩大了事物的稳定性。如果阴阳平衡允许波动的范围较大，它的平衡就不容易被破坏，就有较大的稳定性；如果允许的波动范围较小，它的平衡就比较容易打破，其稳定性就较差；如果允许的波动范围很狭窄，它的平衡就极易被破坏，其稳定性非常不可靠。人体对他所在的周围环境有一种适应能力，就是人体内阴阳平衡所允许的波动范围大小的反映。当周围环境发生了变化，如没有超过人体的适应能力，就不会引起对人体的伤害；如变化超过了人体的适应范围，就要引起对人体的伤害，如冻伤、烧伤、脱水、溺水以及引起感染性疾病的发生。人体适应能力——即阴阳平衡的稳定程度——也就是人体抗御外邪侵袭的能力。

阴阳的平衡是动态的平衡，有两方面的涵义：一是说阴阳平衡是在事物或现象处于不断的运动中求得的；二是说阴阳平衡的平衡位置或平衡范围，在事物或现象的不同运动时期是不相同的，阴阳的平衡位置是随运动而发生变化的。

世界是在不断地运动着的，世界上的事物或现象也是不断地运动着、变化着的。在这种情况下，阴阳只能在运动及变化中来求得平衡，这是动态平衡的第一种涵义。一年四季的周期性变化，引起了气温的周期改变，而人的体温只能控制在 37 ℃左右。因此人体的产热和散热功能就要随四季的变化而发生相应的变化，冬季产热功能加强，夏季散热功能加强，这样才能把人体的体温控制在正常范围之内。又如一个在做自由体操的运动员，他既要作跑、跳、滚、翻等各种动作，又要做出各种姿势，这时如不注意平衡，就要出现失误。在做自由体操时注意平衡，是不同于在静止状态下去注意平衡，是要在每一个动作中，去调整重心、纠正姿势，以维持平衡。在整套动作中，重心要随着动作的需要，时左时右，时高时低，这才能保证动作的准确，姿势的优美，而不至于发生失误。这都说明，运动着的事物或现象，是要在运动中进行自我调节，以求得平衡。

运动中的事物或现象，其阴阳平衡的平衡位置不是固定不变的，而是随着运动变化发生相应的变化，出现涨落变化。一个人从出生到死，经过了生长、成熟、衰老不同的生长时期，这不同时期的实质就是生长和衰老二者之间的平衡。在中年以前，生长居于主导地位，表现为生长、发育，平衡点靠近生长的一侧；到中壮年，生长和衰老基本处于均衡的状态，表现为人在各方面比较成熟，生长和衰老两种趋势均不明显，平衡点是在生长和衰老

50

之间；一旦进入了老年，生长趋势已成强弩之末，衰老趋势正日益增强，而占主导地位，因此，表现以衰老过程为主，则平衡点偏于衰老一侧。所以，从人的一生来看，阴阳的平衡位置，不是固定不变的，而是随着生命的不同时期发生涨落变化，这是动态平衡的第二个涵义。

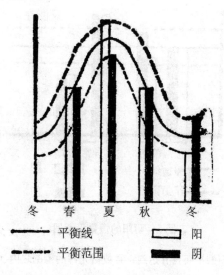

冬　春　夏　秋　冬

━━━　平衡线　　　☐　阳

╌╌╌　平衡范围　　■　阴

图4　阴阳的动态平衡图

说明：图以四季为例说明阴阳的动态平衡。在四季的变化中，阴阳要发生相应的涨落变化，夏至阳气最盛，冬至阴气最盛。因而，阴阳在一年中的波动呈现为双向曲线（如图所示）。而且，阴阳各自都有自己的波动曲线（图中未示），阳气的波动范围，要较阴气波动为大。

阴阳平衡还是一种恒量的平衡（即常数平衡），这是说在一定的时期或阶段，阴阳平衡的范围是个常数，高于或低于这个常数，虽然阴阳是平衡的，也是属于不正常的。只有在常数的范围

51

内，这才是正常的阴阳平衡。如人体内所含的各种成分，都是一个常数。血浆的比重为 1.024～1.029，血液中的红细胞数，男性的为 400～500 万/立方毫米，女性的为 350～450 万/立方毫米。要维持正常的生理功能，人体的各种成分就必须达到正常范围之内。否则，正常生理功能就要受到影响。

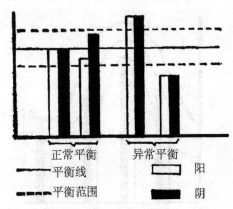

正常平衡　　异常平衡

—————平衡线　　□　阳

-------平衡范围　■　阴

图5　阴阳的恒量平衡图

说明：阴阳的平衡只有达到正常数值允许的范围之内（即阴阳平衡允许的波动范围），才为正常的平衡。在正常数值允许的范围之外，阴阳虽然是平衡的，也是异常的，但为异常的平衡。

人体的阴阳平衡也是这样，必须在常数的范围之内，才是正常的平衡。在不同的年龄阶段，常数的数值是不相同的。但对相同或相近年龄的人来说，常数的数值大致是一样的。阴阳平衡的常数除了和年龄有关外，也和性别有关。由于目前对阴阳尚不能进行定量分析，无从知道各年龄组或性别组阴阳平衡的准确数值，但是，大致上的数量概念还是有的。如临床上所说的阴阳两虚、气血两虚的患者中，就包含有低水平的阴阳平衡在内。他们阴阳虽然是平衡的，但他们还是属于病态。所以在临床治疗中，调理阴阳，"以平为期"，显然是不够的。在治疗中，不仅当使阴阳恢复平衡，而且只有达到正常水平的平衡，才能消除临床上的病态。

阴阳平衡还是一种功能态的平衡，而不一定是数量上的平衡。人是一个生命体，人体内脏腑间的协调，并不是在体积或数量上的相等，而主要是功能上的相当。人体内有的脏器很大，有的却很小，虽然它们在体积上是不相称的，但是它们在功能上却是相当的，都能按时完成维持人体正常生命所需要它完成的任务，因而它们之间是协调的、平衡的。各脏腑、各种物质的功能状态是不一样的，有的作用大，有的作用小，为了要取得功能上的平衡和协调，就不可能在体积或数量方面要求一致。功能上的协调和平衡，比数量或体积上的相等，具有更重要的意义。

要维持阴阳平衡，在自然界或人体内，都存在着一种自动调节的机制，这就是阴阳的对立和制约。

阴阳是一种相对立的概念，对立的双方都能向对方发生制约的作用。阴阳向对方发生制约作用力量的大小，和其本身的盛衰成反比，和对方的盛衰成正比，即在阴阳失去平衡的时候，弱的一方对强的一方施加的制约力量，要比强的一方对弱的一方施加的制约力量要强；而且弱的一方对强者的制约力量是随双方力量的悬殊而增强，强的一方对弱者的制约力量是随双方力量的悬殊而减弱，以致消失。阴阳之间就是通过这种相互制约来维持阴阳平衡。《类经图翼》说："动极者镇之以静，阴亢者胜之以阳。"动到极点（阳亢）则以静（阴）镇之，阴亢则以阳来胜之。"动极"和"阴亢"都是阴阳盛衰的描述，则其对立面必然衰弱到相应的程度。"镇"和"胜"都是对制约力量大小的描述，弱者能对强者施加强大的制约力量。说明了制约力量的大小是和其本身的盛衰成反比，这就是自然界物极必反、垂死挣扎规律的表现，是维持平衡的一种主要方式和手段。

在维护阴阳的平衡中，阴阳的互生也发生一定的作用。阴阳互生的力量和其本身的盛衰成正比。因此，强的一方"生"弱的一方力量强，而弱的一方"生"强的一方力量弱，这也有利于维护阴阳平衡。

阴阳平衡是一种相对的平衡，即阴阳双方总是在平衡允许的范围内，围绕平衡位置进行波动。阴阳的这种波动，就是在阴阳互生和互制这两种力量的作用下产生的，并控制它的波动范围，不超出阴阳平衡允许的波动范围。

人体的体温通过产热和散热这两个过程来进行调节，以维持体温在 37 ℃左右。实际上，体温就是产热（阳）和散热（阴）的平衡点。人体正常的生理活动，包括运动，都要产生热量，以升高人体的温度。同时，人体通过出汗、热的辐射、空气对流来散发体内的热量，以降低体温。产热和散热的共同作用，把人的体温维持在 37 ℃左右。产热和散热可以看作是一对阴阳关系，人的体温则是阴阳的平衡位置，正常体温允许的波动范围，就是阴阳平衡允许的波动范围。为了把阴阳维持在平衡允许的波动范围之内，产热和散热的相互作用，或是互生（共同使体温升高），或是互制（共同把体温降低），协调统一，体温才能正常。在疾病中，由于人体调节体温的功能发生障碍，产热和散热的平衡位置发生偏移，超出了正常体温允许的范围，则要出现体温的升高或降低。如果阴阳调节的机制没有失常，或经过治疗又恢复正常，人体就可以通过阴阳的制约作用，恢复到正常的阴阳平衡，体温也就恢复了正常。

4. 阴阳的运动形式

阴阳之间是对立统一的关系，既相互依存、互生、互根、互用，又相互对立、相互制约、相互斗争，这就引起了阴阳的运动。阴阳的运动形式，就阴阳的相互状态而言，则表现为阴阳的消长变化和阴阳的转化；就事物和它的周围环境的关系而言，则表现为阴阳的升降和出入。

（1）阴阳的消长变化 阴阳平衡是相对的平衡，动态的平衡，是在运动中求得平衡。因而，阴阳平衡在实际中总是围绕一个中心位置（平衡位置）、在一定范围内进行波动。阴阳围绕平衡位置进行的波动变化，即称为阴阳的消长变化，它表现为阴消阳长或阳消阴长。阴阳总是围绕着其平衡位置，在平衡允许的范围内进行波动，它的波动好像潮水一样，一起一伏，一涨一落，波动着向前运动。这种一起一伏的波动，可称为阴阳的"涨落"，一般称为阴阳的消长。消，是消减、衰减的意思；长，是增长的意思。在阴阳的运动中，阴阳总是进行相反方向的运动，即阴涨时阳落，阳涨时阴落，在阴阳的涨落中来维持阴阳的平衡。阴阳的涨落交替进行，这就出现阴消阳长和阳消阴长的交替现象。阴消阳长和阳消阴长连续地进行，这就构成了一个阴阳消长的单位，即消长波。

就自然界而言，春生夏长为阴消阳长，秋收冬藏为阳消阴长，就构成了一年。对植物来说，这就成为一个生长周期。从夜半子时开始的一阳生，到正午阳气盛为阴消阳长，从未时开始的一阴生，到午夜亥时阴气盛为阳消阴长，这个消长波就构成一天，成为年月时间的基础单位。人自出生到壮年，以生长发育为主，衰老只占次要地位，是人身的阴消阳长；从壮年到老年，以衰老为主，生长只占次要地位，是人身的阳消阴长，这个消长波就构成了人的一生。所以，一个消长波是由阴消阳长和阳消阴长两部分构成的，而成为阴阳消长的一个单位。

阴阳消长可以见到两种形式，一种是正常的阴阳消长，一种是异常的阴阳消长。

正常的阴阳消长是符合自然界发展的一般规律。正常的阴阳消长具备以下两个特点：一是阴阳消长所表现的涨落变化，只在阴阳平衡允许的范围内进行；二是在阴阳消长的过程中，包含阴消阳长和阳消阴长两个过程，构成了一个完整的消长波。在消长过程中，每一个具体的点上，阴阳虽然是不平衡的，但在总体上阴阳是平衡的。

如以一年中白昼和黑夜的长短来讨论阴阳的消长关系，白昼为阳，黑夜为阴。冬至以后白昼逐渐增长，黑夜逐渐缩短，一直到夏至这一天，白昼时间最长，白昼比黑夜长出 6 小时 12 分钟（根据呼和浩特计时）。夏至以后白昼缩短，黑夜增长，直至冬至这天，黑夜时间最长，要比白昼长出 5 小时 22 分钟（根据呼和浩特计时）。由冬至到夏至，白昼增长，黑夜缩短，故为阴消阳长；从夏至到冬至，白昼缩短，黑夜增长，故为阳消阴长。在一年之中，只有春分和秋分两天白昼与黑夜基本相等。在春分至秋分这半年中，白昼均长于黑夜，为阳盛；从秋分到春分的半年中，黑夜均长于白昼，为阴盛。而夏至这一天白昼最长，黑夜最短，为阳极；冬至黑夜最长，白昼最短，为阴极。白昼和黑夜的波动范围几乎达 12 小时，虽然波动范围如此之大，但这属于正常现象。所以，这就是一年之中阴阳平衡（白昼与黑夜间的平衡）允许的波动范围。虽然一年中 365 天的白昼与黑夜长短不等，但从总体来看，白昼和黑夜基本上各占一半时间。所以，在整体上阴阳是平衡的。

阴阳消长发生的机制是阴阳互生和互制双重作用的结果。在阴阳消长的过程中，由于阴阳中的一方不断增长，而它的对立面则不断消减。增长的一方随着它的增长，它对对方的互生作用不断加强，而制约作用则不断削弱，因而导致它的对立面由消减转化为增长；阴阳中消减的一方随着它的消减，它对对方的制约作用不断增强，而相生作用则不断消弱，终于导致它的对立面由增长转化为消减。这种互生互制作用控制了阴阳双方不能远离阴阳的平衡位置，只能围绕平衡位置在阴阳平衡允许的范围内进行涨落变化。

异常的阴阳消长是指阴阳的消长不符合自然界发展的一般规律，它破坏了阴阳的平衡，导致了事物的消亡，在人体则表现为病理状态，异常的阴阳消长也具备两个特点：一是阴阳消长超出了阴阳平衡允许的波动范围，朝着远离平衡位置的方向运动，终于导致阴阳平衡的破坏，事物或现象失去了稳定状态；二是异常的阴阳消长不能构成一个完整的阴阳消长波，或只有阴消阳长的过程，或只有阳消阴长的过程，最终导致阳盛阴衰或阴盛阳衰，引起了阴阳离决。从整个过程来看，由于不能构成一个完整的消长波，所以阴阳不可能平衡。

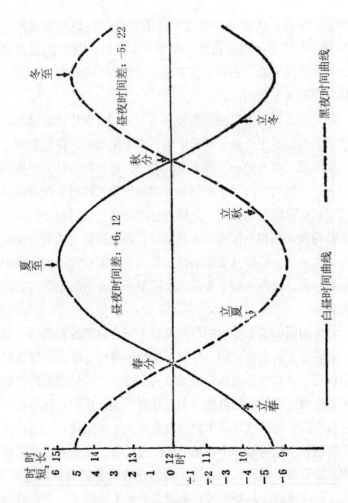

图6 呼和浩特地区昼夜时差曲线图

说明：在坐标图中，纵坐标表示时间（以小时为单位），左侧数值表示昼夜时差。右侧数值表示昼夜的时长。横坐标表示四季的变化。图中实线为白昼曲线，即阳气的消长；虚线为黑夜曲线，即阴气的消长。夏至，白昼比黑夜长 6 时 12 分；冬至，白昼比黑夜短 5 时 22 分。在一年中，夏至为阳盛之极，冬至为阴盛之极，为一年中两个阴阳的转化点。通过夏至或冬至两个时间，阴阳的升降发生逆转。其他时间均为阴阳消长，只有升降速度的变化，升降不发生逆转。在图中可以看出，阴阳转化是间断性的，以突变的形式出现，有明确的方向性，即总是指向阴阳平衡的中心线；阴阳消长是连续性的，以渐变的形式出现，方向性不明确，即在未通过阴阳平衡的中心线时，是指向中心线，通过中心线后，是指向远离中心线的方向。

异常的阴阳消长在人体上，只见于疾病之中。一个外感风热的病人，由于阳邪所伤，而致阳气亢盛。开始只是阳盛而阴未伤，随后损伤阴气，而致阳盛阴虚。如果未经恰当的治疗，病情进一步恶化，使阳气越来越盛，阴气越来越虚，最后必致阳极而阴竭。阴竭于内，阴不为阳之"守"，阳也不为阴之"用"，阳气亡越于外，终致阴阳离决，引起死亡。

异常阴阳消长发生的原因，一是阴阳互生互制作用发生异常，阴阳互制的力量和阴阳本身的盛衰成正比，阴阳互生的力量则和阴阳本身的盛衰成反比，出现了以强凌弱的现象。使强者益强，弱者越弱，阴阳各自向远离阴阳平衡位置的方向发展，而不能趋向于平衡，终于导致阴阳的离决。由于异常的阴阳消长是向远离阴阳平衡的方向发展，所以，它不可能构成一个完整的阴阳消长波。

异常的阴阳消长还可以是在外因的作用下发生的。虽然阴阳的互生互制功能并未异常，但是外加的力量超过了阴阳本身具有的调节能力，导致阴阳消长朝着远离阴阳平衡的方向发展。在这种情况下，只要外加力量一有削弱或外邪被祛除，阴阳就可以通过自身的调节，使失去的平衡重新建立。

（2）阴阳的转化　阴阳运动到一定程度，阴阳各自向其对立面发生转化，即阴转化为阳或阳转化为阴，这就称为阴阳转化。

阴阳转化不同于阴阳消长，它有四个特点：一是阴阳转化要引起阴阳的属性发生变化，也就是包含有"质变"的意思；二是阴阳转化的发生是有条件的，不是任何时候都可以发生的，三是阴阳转化是间断出现的，是以突变的形式出现的；四是阴阳转化是有方向性的，是朝着阴阳平衡的位置发生转化。

阴阳转化要引起阴阳的属性发生变化，即阴转变为阳，阳转变为阴。而阴阳消长只引起数量方面的变化，阴还是阴，阳还是阳，在阴阳属性上并无变化，从一年阴阳消长的曲线图中可以看出：冬至开始阳气生，白昼逐渐增长，黑夜逐渐缩短，一直延续到夏至；夏至开始阴气生，白昼逐渐缩短，黑夜逐渐增长，一直延续到冬至。从冬至到夏至为阴消阳长，从曲线上显示出，开始变化较慢，而后几乎呈直线上升，之后又变为缓慢；从夏至到冬至为阳消阴长，从曲线上显示出，开始曲线平坦，而后几乎呈直线下降，之后曲线又较平坦。这些说明，阴阳消长过程中，只有数量方面的变化，而无"质"的变化。夏至和冬至是一年中两个阴阳转化点，夏至以前是阴消阳长，夏至后则是阳消阴长；冬至以前是阳消阴长，冬至后则是阴消阳长。通过夏至和冬至这两个节气，阴阳消长发生了逆转。通过夏至，阳气由升变为降：通过冬至，阳气由降变为升。升为阳，降为阴，所以，经过夏至，阳转化为阴，经过冬至，则阴转化为阳。这说明事物的性质发生了变化。所以，阴阳转化是要引起阴阳的属性发生变化，它包含着"质"的变化，有"质变"的含义。

阴阳转化的发生是有条件的，在《内经》中讨论到阴阳转化时，常用"重""极""甚"三字来表示发生转化的条件，"重""极""甚"三字的意义是相同的，都表示"顶点""严重""极点"等意思，说明只有在运动或变化发展到极点时，才能发生阴阳转化。在一年中只有在夏至和冬至两个节气，才发生阴阳转化。夏至是阳盛之极，冬至是阴盛之极。阳盛之极，必然转化为它的对立面——阴；阴盛之极，也必然转化为它的对立面——阳。在人体上，当生长发育已经达到极点时，即开始迈向衰老，这也是阴阳转化。而阴阳消长则不同，随时都在进行，因而是无条件的。

　　一年中，阴阳转化只发生在夏至和冬至两个节气，而不是连续发生的，是间断的，是突然发生的，而且经常是在瞬间结束。所以，阴阳转化常以"突变"的形式出现。阴阳转化的开始，也就是它的结束，是在短促的时间内完成。阴阳消长则不同，它是连续地进行，是在相当长的时间内逐渐地进行，直至引起了阴阳转化，它又开始了反方向的阴阳消长。所以，阴阳消长是连续不断的，是逐渐发生的，是以一种"渐变"的形式表现出来，常看不到它的结束，看到的只是消长的形式有所变化。

　　阴阳转化是有方向性的，即在正常情况下的阴阳转化，它的方向总是指向阴阳的平衡位置。当阴阳消长达到极限时，也即达到了阴阳平衡允许的波动范围的边缘时，如果再进一步消长，必然破坏阴阳的平衡。阴阳转化就在这时间发生，它使阴阳消长的方向发生逆转，指向阴阳平衡的位置。阴阳消长则不同，当阴阳消长尚未通过阴阳的平衡位置时，阴阳消长的方向是指向阴阳的平衡位置；阴阳消长一旦通过了阴阳平衡的位置，则阴阳消长的方向，则是指向远离平衡的位置。可以认为，阴阳消长似乎类似于"惯性"运动，所以说，阴阳消长的方向并不永远指向阴阳平衡的位置，而是靠阴阳转化的调整，它才不致破坏阴阳平衡。所以说，从阴阳的运动形式而言，阴阳转化的目的是明确的，总是趋向于阴阳平衡，是阴阳维护其平衡的主要运动形式。

阴阳转化是采用"突变"的形式表现出来的。而"突变"的发生过程，也有两种形式。一般地说，阴阳转化总是和阴阳消长相连续，它是在阴阳消长进行的基础上发生的。例如夏至和冬至发生的阴阳转化，它是阴阳消长进行到一定程度的必然结果。人的正常死亡（老死）和一般因病而死者，在死亡前均有相应的阴阳消长变化。只有阴阳消长达到一定程度，才能引起死亡。这些阴阳转化"突变"的发生，都是阴阳消长"渐变"的必然结果，符合自然界的一般规律。但是，阴阳转化有时并不和阴阳消长相连续，不是在阴阳消长进行的基础上发生的，而是独立发生的。例如地震、山洪或其他偶然遇上的意外事故造成了人和生物的突然死亡，就其个体而言，其本身的阴阳消长还未达到足以引起阴阳转化（死亡）的程度，它和阴阳消长没有任何的关系，完全是一种偶然的巧合。

阴阳转化是阴阳互制和互生作用的结果。根据阴阳互制和制约者的盛衰成反比、和被制约者的盛衰成正比，阴阳互生和相生者盛衰成正比、和被生者盛衰成反比的原理，在阴阳消长过程中，当衰减的一方衰减到阴阳平衡允许波动范围的最低限度时，它必然要向对立面发生强大的制约作用，而相生作用则减弱到最小的程度，迫使对立面发生逆转运动，由增长转变为衰减；当增长的一方增长到阴阳平衡允许波动范围的最高限度时，它向对立面施加的制约作用已减弱到最小程度，而相生作用则增强到最大程度，促使对立面发生逆转运动，由衰减转变为增长，在阴阳消长过程中，增长的一方转变为衰减，衰减的一方转变为增长，使已经远离阴阳平衡的阴阳消长发生逆转，趋向于阴阳平衡的位置，这就是阴阳转化。

当阴阳相互制约功能失常时，失去了对阴阳消长的控制作用，不能使远离阴阳平衡的消长发生逆转，甚至发生相反的作用，这就要引起异常的阴阳消长和异常的阴阳转化，在人体上，这只见于病理状态下。

（3）阴阳消长和阴阳转化的辩证关系　阴阳消长和阴阳转化是阴阳的两种运动形式，都是由于阴阳的互生和互制引起的，共同构成了阴阳完整的运动状态。使阴阳处于不断的运动之中，维持了阴阳的平衡，也就维持了事物或现象的稳定状态。阴阳消长和阴阳转化共存于一体之中，相互为用，相互制约，它们本身就是一对阴阳关系。

一般地说，阴阳转化是在阴阳消长的基础上发生的，只有当阴阳消长进行到一定程度，必然地要发生阴阳转化。如阴阳消长进行到一定程度，仍不发生阴阳转化，出现过度的阴阳消长，就必然导致阴阳平衡被破坏。阴阳消长的限度，就是阴阳转化发生的条件，也就是阴阳平衡允许的最大波动范围。在这范围内的阴阳波动，不足以危害阴阳平衡；波动超出了范围，必然导致阴阳平衡的破坏。

阴阳消长是在低一层次阴阳转化的基础上发生的。任何事物的结构均具有层次性，高一层次的结构是由低一层次结构构成的，低一层次结构又是更低层次结构所构成的，这就形成了事物的层次性。每一层次结构均有自己结构的完整性，功能上的全面性，并成为相对独立的单位，在一定条件下能够独立存在。上一层次的阴阳消长，实际上就是下一层次阴阳转化的结果。由于下一层次各组成单位有序地发生阴阳转化，阴转化为阳，则在上一层次表现出阴消阳长；阳转化为阴，则在上一层次表现出阳消阴长。这就是阴阳消长和阴阳转化的互用关系。阴阳转化限制了阴阳消长的范围，使阴阳消长不至于无限制地进行下去，维护了阴阳平衡；阴阳消长把阴阳转化割裂开来，使阴阳转化不至于连续不断地发生，使事物发展呈现出阶段性，能有相对的稳定阶段，这就是阴阳消长和阴阳转化的互制关系。

阴阳消长和阴阳转化间的互用和互制，就是二者之间对立统一的辩证关系。

5. 阴阳的升降出入

一个事物包含了阴和阳两个组成部分，阴阳也表示了事物的整体性，即构成了相对独立的单位。

一个相对独立的整体，阴阳在其内部进行着永不停止的运动，这就引起了阴阳的消长和转化。阳主升，阴主降；阳在上，阴在下。在上之阳必然下交于阴，这是由于阴气下吸之故；在下之阴必须上交于阳，这是由于阳气上蒸之故。阳气下降，阴气上升，引起了阴阳的升降运动，导致了阴阳的消长和转化，促成了事物的生长壮老已和生长化收藏的变化。

任何一个事物，它虽然是相对完整的和独立的，但它总是生活在具体的环境之中，是这个环境的组成部分之一。因而，它既要对周围环境发生作用，周围环境也要对它发生作用。所以，在阴阳的体系中，阴阳永远不是封闭的系统，而是开放的系统，它要和外界发生千丝万缕的联系。例如一个人要从外界摄取饮食和空气等，又要向外界排出人体所不需要的各种废物，与外界进行物质交换。同时，外界的任何变化，都要对人体发生作用；人体的任何变化，也要对周围环境产生作用。由于阴阳是个开放系统，所以它必然和外界交换物质和信息，这就是阴阳的出入运动。所以《素问·六微旨大论》说："故非出入，则无以生长壮老已；非升降，则无以生长化收藏。是以升降出入，无器不有。"

6. 从"太极图"看阴阳学说

"太极图"是古人对阴阳学说的概括，它包含了阴阳学说的主要内容。现就"太极图"来对阴阳学说作一概括的说明。"太极图"是一个圆形的图，中间用一条"～"形的曲线将圆平分为二，而成为蝌蚪状的两部分，被称为"阴阳鱼"。"阴阳鱼"中大的一端为头部，尖端为尾部，两部分别用黑白二色涂抹，以示阴阳。在黑色"阴阳鱼"的头部有一白色的小点，在白色"阴阳鱼"的头部有一黑色的小点，称为"小心"或"眼"，这就构成了一幅"太极图"。

（1）"太极图"是一个圆形，分成黑白两部分，黑者为阴，白色为阳，阴阳共存于一圆之中，说明了阴阳存在于一体之中和阴阳的整体性。

（2）在图中，阴阳两部分的面积是相等的，说明了阴阳是平衡的。

（3）圆中，用"～"形的曲线将圆平分，而不用直线来平分，以表示阴阳是处于不断的运动之中。

（4）在图中，白色"阴阳鱼"头部有黑色的"小心"，黑

65

色"阴阳鱼"头部有白色的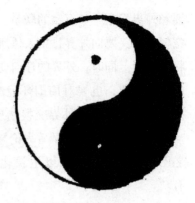
"小心",说明了阴中有阳,阳
中有阴,阴阳是不可分的,阴阳
是互根的。

(5)通过阴阳各自的"小
心"和大圆的圆心的直线,既是
大圆的直径,也是阴阳两部分各
自小圆的直径,为阴阳各自的极
点。阴阳的转化也就是从这一直
线的两端开始的,即阴极生阳,

图7 太极图

阳极生阴。说明了阴阳的转化是有条件的,当阴阳消长发展到极
点时,才能引起阴阳的转化。

(6)阴阳转化是从通过圆心阴阳两部"小心"直线的两端
开始的,阴阳各自向其对立面发生转化,即阴转化为阳,阳转化
为阴。所以,在阴阳的运动中,"阴阳鱼"的头部是向后回缩
的,其尾部则是向前运动,共同围绕着"太极图"的圆心,进
行圆周运动,这就表现为阴阳的升降运动。

(7)通过"太极图"的圆心所作的任何一条直径,把"太
极图"分为两个半圆。任何一个半圆中的阴阳两部分,除在特
殊情况下,都是不相等的。这说明在具体的事物中,阴阳总是不
平衡的;但从整体来看,阴阳却是平衡的。整体的阴阳平衡,正
是建立在具体的阴阳不平衡的基础之上的。

(8)通过"太极图"的圆心所作的任何一条直径,把"太
极图"分为两个半圆。任何一个半圆中,必然包含着阴阳两个
部分。说明了任何事物或现象,都是由阴阳两部分所构成的,纯

66

阴或纯阳所构成的事物，在实际上是不存在的。

（9）一个"太极图"可以看作是无数小太极图所构成的。
"太极图"的阴阳消长正是这些无数小"太极图"阴阳转化的结
果。而"太极图"其本身的阴阳转化，又是其本身阴阳消长达
到极点时发生的。所以说，阴阳转化是同层次阴阳消长的结果，
阴阳消长又是低层次阴阳转化的结果。说明了阴阳转化和阴阳消
长是互根互制的。

（三）阴阳学说在医学上的应用

阴阳学说是中医学理论的指导思想和方法论，它贯穿于中医
学的各个方面，对人与自然的关系，人体的生理、病理、药物的
作用，临床上的诊断和治疗等，都要用阴阳学说作为指导，应用
阴阳学说的方法，来分析和处理问题。

1. 使人与自然的关系具体化

天地有阴阳，人体也分阴阳，天地之阴阳与人体之阴阳相呼
应。这就为"天人一体""天人相应"的理论提供了理论根据。

春夏阳升，秋冬阴长，这是一年四季中阴阳的消长变化。在
自然界的生物中，就引起了春生夏长、秋收冬藏的变化，在人体
也发生相应的变化。在这基础上就提出春夏养阳、秋冬养阴的养
生补虚的思想。

在一天中，子时一阳生，午时阳盛，未时一阴生，亥时阴
盛。一天阴阳升降的变化要引起人体发生相应的变化。这为临床
上的诊断以及判断经气的循行、腧穴的开合提供了理论依据。临
床上对阴阳盛衰的判断、针灸上按时取穴等，均以此为据。

2. 建立人体生理学理论

（1）对人体结构阴阳属性的分析　对人体结构的阴阳分析，

大体上是根据上下、内外等来进行。如以人体而言，腰以上为阳，腰以下为阴；体表为阳，体内为阴；六腑为阳，五脏为阴；五脏中以心肺为阳，肝脾肾为阴等。腰以上为阳，故风热阳邪多从上受；腰以下为阴，故寒湿阴邪多从下受。体表为阳，故六淫之邪多从外受；体内为阴，故饮食、劳倦、七情等邪皆从内受。六腑为阳，故六腑的功能以传导化物为主，以通为用，六腑之病多属热证、实证；五脏属阴，故五脏的功能以贮藏精气为主，以藏为用，五脏之病多属寒证、虚证。心肺为阳，一属火一主气，而主气血，故心肺之病可见阳热之证；肝脾肾属阴，而主精血，故肝脾肾之病更多见到的属虚证，或为寒证。

由于人体组织结构的阴阳属性不同，因而在生理上及病理上均有差别，为临床的诊断和治疗提供了根据。

（2）建立生理学的理论　在阴阳学说的指导下，结合人体的具体情况，建立了人体生理学理论。

以阴阳学说建立起来的生理学理论，都采用了两分法的方法：人体的脏腑以脏为阴、腑为阳，脏主藏而腑主化；就每个脏腑而言，均有阴阳、气血，阴血主滋养濡润，阳气主温煦鼓动；就整体而言，除阴阳、气血外，还有营卫、津液。这些脏腑、气血、营卫、津液等，实际是阴阳两分法的表现。因此，它们二者之间均是相反相成，都是一组阴阳关系，共同完成它们的生理功能。

"气化"是指人体内物质或能量的转化，生命赖以维持。"气化"是在气的"升降出入"过程中发生的，《素问·六微旨大论》说："气之升降，天地之更用也……天气下降，气流于地；地气上升，气腾于天。故高下相召，升降相因，而变作矣。"气的升降，是天地相互作用的结果。天气下降，作用于地；地气上升，作用于天。正是由于天地之气的相交，因而引起万物的变化，生命也赖以产生并维持。天地之气的相交，实际就是阴阳之气的相交。所以，"气化"也是由于阴阳的"升降"引起的。就人体而言，"升降"是指人体内气的运动形式，"出入"是指人体和外界进行的物质交换。《素问·六微旨大论》说："出入废则神机化灭，升降息则气立孤危。""出入"停止了，人体不再和外界进行物质交换，生命就不能维持；"升降"停止了，气也就难以再存在了。这就说明了气的运动和"气化"在生命中的重要性。实际上，这就是用阴阳学说对生命现象的具体说明。

阴阳平衡、阴阳消长、阴阳转化，这都是中医生理学的基本观点，中医生理学理论就建立在这些基础之上。

3. 建立病理学理论

（1）对于病因的认识　在《内经》中，已采用阴阳的观点来认识致病因素。它认为气候变化而产生的致病因素，如风雨寒暑等是从皮肤侵入人体，经经络而内传于脏腑；而其他如精神性致病因素、饮食因素等，则是内伤脏腑。所以《素问·调经论》说："夫邪之生也，或生于阴，或生于阳。其生于阳者，得之风雨寒暑；其生于阴者，得之饮食居处，阴阳喜怒。"《内经》还把同是外邪的风雨寒湿，按其属性又分阴阳两类，认为属天气所化的风雨，所致之病为实；由地气所化的寒湿，所致之病为虚。

（2）建立病理学理论　阴阳的平衡和协调是中医生理学理论的基础，是维持人体正常生理功能的先决条件。而阴阳平衡的丧失，阴阳失调则是中医病理学的基石。

阴阳平衡的失调，可以是在外邪的作用下，破坏了阴阳平衡引起的；也可以是脏腑功能失常的结果。

外邪有阴阳的不同，作用于人体则能引起阴阳的盛衰。

《素问·阴阳应象大论》说："阴胜则阳病，阳胜则阴病。阳胜则热，阴胜则寒。"这常是在外邪作用下，而导致人体阴阳失调的表现。"阴胜则阳病""阴胜则寒"，这常由外感阴寒之邪所致，导致阴寒偏盛，阳气偏衰，阳气温煦功能失常，所以出现寒象；"阳胜则阴病""阳胜则热"，是由外感温热阳邪所致，使阳气偏盛，阴气耗伤，阴气不能制阳，所以出现热象。由外邪所引起的阴阳偏盛之证，其亢盛的一面是主要的，而不足的一面是相对的。所以，这类疾病多属实证。

脏腑功能失调，多由七情、饮食、劳倦、房室等因素所致，它直接作用于脏腑，引起脏腑、阴阳、气血的紊乱，导致阴阳、气血的偏衰。阴虚则相对"阳盛"，"阳盛则热"，出现虚热之证，所以说"阴虚则热"；阳虚则相对"阴盛"，"阴盛则寒"，出现虚寒之证，所以说"阳虚则寒"。

由于阴阳互根，阴阳有互生作用。所以，当阴阳中之一方，由于虚甚而不能互生，则必然要累及它的对立面，导致阴阳两虚。这即所说的"阴损及阳""阳损及阴"的病理过程。

在疾病的过程中，还可以引起阴阳间的制约发生障碍，导致阴阳消长的异常，这就加重了阴阳的失调。当阴阳消长达到一个"极限"的水平时，就可以引起阴阳的转化，《素问·阴阳应象大论》说："重寒则热，重热则寒。""重阴必阳，重阳必阴。"说明了寒甚之极，可以出现"热"象；热甚之极，也可以出现"寒"象，甚至热证还可以转化为寒证。虚证之极可以出现

"实"象，实证之极可以出现"虚"象。这些都是由阴阳转化引起来的。但是，由热证转化为寒证、实证转化为虚证，这是疾病恶化的必然结果；而寒证出现"热"象、虚证出现"实"象，这都是一种假象，不是疾病好转的表现，而是疾病恶化的结果。总之，这些经常是在病情危重时才出现的表现。

4. 在临床诊断上的应用

疾病的发生是由阴阳失调引起的，所以，在诊断疾病时，辨别阴阳就显得更重要了。《素问·阴阳应象大论》说："善诊者，察色按脉，先别阴阳。"

"先别阴阳"，可以有两层含意，一是辨别症状的阴阳属性，二是辨别阴证阳证。

辨别症状的阴阳属性，这是"四诊"中的任务之一，一是根据色泽的明暗来分辨阴阳，色泽鲜明者病在阳分，多为实证、热证；色泽晦暗者，病在阴分，多为虚证、寒证。二是从声音来辨别阴阳，声音高亢洪亮，多言躁动，多属实证、热证；声音低弱无力，少言安静，多属虚证、寒证。三是从脉象中来辨别阴阳，凡是浮大数洪之脉为阳；凡是沉细迟弱者为阴。在四诊中辨别阴阳，就为辨别阴证和阳证提供了依据。

在辨证时，首先是进行"八纲"辨证，即辨表里、虚实、寒热、阴阳。其中阴阳是总纲，表里是辨病位，寒热是辨病性，虚实是辨邪正的相互状态。辨疾病的部位，即辨疾病是在表还是在里，或在何脏何腑；辨疾病的性质，即是辨病证的属性，是寒、是热、是燥、是湿；辨邪正相互的状态，即是辨别属虚、属实，以及虚实的多少。以上辨别明确后，凡属表证、热证、实证即为阳证；里证、寒证、虚证为阴证。就一般而言，表、实、热证为典型的阳证，里、虚、寒证为典型的阴证。

5. 指导临床治疗

《素问·阴阳应象大论》说："谨察阴阳所在而调之，以平为期。"说明调理阴阳、恢复阴阳平衡，是中医治疗的基本原则。

调理阴阳的方法，就是根据阴阳的盛衰而进行调理，当"损其有余，补其不足""实则泻之，虚则补之"。

对于阴阳偏盛者，当"损其有余"。"阳盛则热"，故对阳盛者，当以寒药折其过甚之阳。"阴盛则寒"，故对阴盛者，则以温热之剂，折其过盛之阴寒。对于阴阳偏衰者，当"补其不足"。"阳虚则寒"，故当以温热之品以补其不足之阳气。"阴虚则热"，故当以甘寒之品，滋其阴而除其热。

在对阴阳进行调补时，必须注意阴阳互根的原理。张景岳说："善补阳者，必于阴中求阳，则阳得阴助而生化无穷；善补阴者，必于阳中求阴，则阴得阳升而源泉不竭。"在补阳时，必须同时佐以补阴之品；在补阴时，又当佐以补阳之品，以使阴阳得以互化。

二、五行学说

五行学说和阴阳学说一样，也是我国古代具有朴素唯物论和辩证法思想的哲学理论，它曾经在历史上占有重要地位。

（一）五行概念的形成

"五行"概念的形成很早，至少在商周之时已经产生。

"五行"概念是古人在生活中形成的。古人发现木、火、土、金、水这五种物质，是人们生活所不可缺少的。于是产生了

72

"五材"的概念。《左传》说:"天生五材,民并用之,废一不可。"自然界给我们产生了五种材料,老百姓都加以应用,缺少一样也是不行的。《尚书》也说:"水火者,百姓之所饮食也;金木者,百姓之所兴作也;土者,万物之所资生也,是为人用。"水、火是百姓饮食之所必需的,金、木是百姓劳动兴建所依赖的,土是百姓赖以生存的,万物都靠土来生长,这些都是被人们所利用的。

"五材"的概念是从人们生活的需要提出来的,是人们生活所必不可缺少的基本物质。

木、火、土、金、水是人们生活所必需的,人们日常的用具是由这些物质制成的。如生活中用的瓦罐,就是用土加水制成后,再用火烧制而成;房屋就是用木、土、水三者制成;打猎或耕作用的工具,则是由木和金制作而成。根据这些事例,古人进一步推想,自然界的万物也是由这五种基本物质所构成的。正如《国语》所说:"故先王以土与金、木、水、火杂以成百物。"所以,早先的圣贤,用土和金、木、水、火揉合在一起而制成各种各样的东西。这样就把木、火、土、金、水当成构成自然界万物的"元素",这显然是解释不通的,把具体物质变成一种抽象的属性,似乎更合理一些。所以《尚书·洪范》说:"水曰润下,火曰炎上,木曰曲直,金曰从革,土爰稼穑。"水具有滋润和下流的特性,火具有温热和上升的特性,木具有曲直生长的特性,金具有容易变化的特性,土具有生长庄稼的特性。从五种具体物质中抽出它们的特性,作为木、火、土、金、水的涵义,这样,"五行"就由具体的物质变成只表示这五种属性的抽象概念。到这时候,哲学上的"五行"概念才算初步形成。"五"是指木、火、土、金、水这五种属性；"行"是这五种属性间运动变化的规律性。"五行学说"认为世界上的事物或现象，其内部都包含有木、火、土、金、水这五种属性，这五种属性间的相互关系（即相互的联系方式和运动状态）决定了事物或现象的发生和发展；事物或现象之间的差异性，就是由这五种属性间的运动状态所规定的。

到了战国末期，经过邹衍"推演五行"，把精气学说、阴阳学说和五行学说揉合为一体，创立了阴阳五行学说，这才使五行学说的理论更为完善。

（二）五行学说的基本内容

五行学说的基本内容包括五行归类法，五行生克制化和五行乘侮。

1. 五行归类法

五行归类法是以五行所代表的属性为依据，把自然界的事物或现象的某一属性和它类比，从而归属于木、火、土、金、水五大类之中，形成五个大系统。

五行所代表的属性，是从木、火、土、金、水五种具体物质中提取出来的。

木的特性：木包括所有的草木在内。它生长的特点是枝干曲直，尽量向上、向外舒展，以争取获得更多的阳光，为生存取得良好的条件；它枝条柔软，极易弯曲，又易复原；它有很强的生命能力，只要有一定的条件，就能顽强地生存下去。古人把木的特性归纳为：生发、柔和、曲直、舒展等。

火的特性：火在燃烧时的特点是温热、光亮、火苗向上，并能引起空气向上流动。古人把火的特性归纳为：炎上、阳热、升腾等。

土的特性：土承受了万物，万物皆生于土，这说明土中包含有万物生长的必要因素。万物埋于土中，能被腐蚀而消失。古人把土的特性归纳为：长养、生化、受纳、变化等。

金的特性：人类最早发现的金属是锡，而后是铜。说金色白，是根据锡而言。金属的特点，一是导热性良，所以给人以清凉的感觉；二是不易被污染，即使有污染，一擦一洗即去；三是金属的比重大，给人以沉重之感；四是金属坚硬而富有韧性，五是金属得火之炼则化，可以任意铸形。古人把金的特性归纳为：清凉、洁净、肃降，收敛等。

水的特性：水为液体，总向下流。水能湿物，使之润泽而不燥。水性本寒，其能灭火，即使炎热的暑天，井中之水也寒冷刺骨。古人把水的特性归纳为：寒湿、下行、滋润等。

五行学说认为，世界是由具有木、火、土、金、水五种属性的物质所构成的。所以，世界上的万物或现象都可以根据"五行"的属性归类。如一年可以分为春、夏、长夏、秋、冬"五季"；气候变化可以分成风、暑、湿、燥、寒"五气"；方位可以分为东、南、中、西、北"五方"；颜色可以分为苍（青）、赤（红）、黄、白、黑"五色"；生物的生命过程可以分为生、长、化、收、藏"五化"；气味可以分为酸、苦、甘、辛、咸"五味"；一天可以分为平旦、日中、日西、合夜、夜半"五时"；人体有肝、心、脾、肺、肾"五脏"，胆、小肠、胃、大肠、膀胱"五腑"，筋、脉、肌肉、皮毛、骨"五体"，目、舌、口、鼻、耳"五官"，魂、神、意、魄、志"五神"，怒、喜、思、悲、恐"五志"等。

以上的五季、五气、五化以及人体上的五脏、五官等，都可以通过属性类比的方法而归属木、火、土、金、水五类之中。如木有生发的特性，而春季为草木萌发，是生长周期的开始，生机勃勃，故春属木类；草木萌发，大地返青，故青色属木；我国东方临海，风调雨顺，气候温暖潮湿，适宜植物的生长，故东方属木；生是生长过程的开始，生机旺盛，故生属木；果实未熟之前，其味多酸，故酸属木；平旦是一日的开始，太阳是从东方升起，是阳气升发之时，故平旦属木。通过这样推理演绎，进行类比，把春、风、青、东方、生、酸、平旦等归属于木类。结合到人体，肝脏的功能以疏泄气机为特点，性喜条达，故属于木。胆与肝为表里，胆附于肝；肝主筋，筋赖肝养；肝开窍于目，肝气和则目能辨黑白；肝藏魂；肝主怒。所以在人体中，把肝、胆、筋、目、魂、怒等归属木类。

五行归类简表

五行	五行属性	五季	五方	五化	五色	五味	五气	五时	五音	五谷	五畜	五脏	五腑	五体
木	生发舒展	春	东	生	苍	酸	风	平旦	角	麻	犬	肝	胆	筋
火	温热炎上	夏	南	长	赤	苦	暑	日中	徵	麦	马	心	小肠	脉
土	长养变化	长夏	中	化	黄	甘	湿	日西	宫	稷	牛	脾	胃	肌肉
金	清肃收敛	秋	西	收	白	辛	燥	合夜	商	稻	鸡	肺	大肠	皮毛
水	寒湿下行	冬	北	藏	黑	咸	寒	夜半	羽	豆	豕	肾	膀胱	骨

自然界或人体之所以可以用五行的属性进行分类，其前提就在于自然界是一个整体，人体也是个整体，而且上面所列举的季节、方位、气候、生命过程、颜色、昼夜、味道以及人体的脏、腑、形体、官窍、神志、情志等，各自都可以构成一个相对独立的整体。五行归类法只适用于对相对独立的整体进行分析和归类。不能构成为一个整体的事物或现象，就不能采用这一方法。

2. 五行的生克制化

五行学说不仅是一种分类方法，更重要的它是阐明事物内部运动一般性规律的学说。事物总是可分的，总是由几部分构成的，其构成部分之间总是要以一定的方式发生联系，并要不停地运动，五行学说就是用"生克制化"的理论来阐明维持事物内部各构成部分之间的平衡和协调，即维持事物的整体性、统一性和稳定性的具体方式。

古人把事物间的各种联系方式概括为"互利"和"互害"两种关系。在五行学说中把"互利"关系称为"相生"，把"互害"关系称为"相克"。"相生"是表示事物间相互资助、相互养育、相互促进的关系，即互生、互助、互根、互用的关系；"相克"是表示事物间相互克制、相互制约、相互对立、相互斗争和相互控制的关系。五行学说用"相生"和"相克"的关系来说明五行间的联系方式，来说明事物或现象内部维持平衡和协调的机制。

五行的"生克"有正常的和异常的。五行学说把事物间正常的"生克"称之为"生克"，把异常的"生克"称之为"乘侮"。

（1）五行的生克　五行的"生克"即指五行"相生"和五

行"相克"，它是指五行间正常的相互资生和相互克制的关系。

五行"相生"有一定的顺序，即按木、火、土、金、水的顺序依次相互资生，即木生火、火生土、土生金、金生水、水生木。

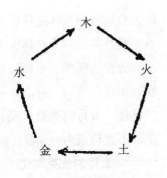

图8　五行相生图

五行"相生"的顺序根据是古人对自然现象的观察得出来的。如钻木能取火，树枝能引火，所以认为木能生火；物被火焚而成灰，灰即是土，故火能生土；金属是从矿石中提炼出来的，矿石又是从土底下开采出来的，是埋藏于地下的，古人认为是由土变化而成的，所以土能生金；水气易在光滑的金属表面凝结成水珠，且在山多之处常多雾气，山必有石，石多有矿，山石洞中每是潮湿润泽，滴水涌泉，古人认为这些水气是由金气所化生，故金能生水；草木虽是生长于土中，但是干旱之地草木并不能生长，必须得到水的湿润后方能生长，所以认为水能生木。《难经》把五行的"相生"关系称为"母子"关系；以"生"我者为"母"，我"生"者为"子"。故对"木"而言，水生木，水为木之"母"；木生火，火为木之"子"。五行"相克"也是按一定顺序进行的，若以木、火、土、金、水的顺序，则相间为"克"，即木克土、土克水、水克火、火克金、金克木。

五行"相克"的顺序也是古人从对自然现象的观察中归纳出来的。土再结实，草木总是能够生长的，一经草木生长，土质也就变得松软了，草木之根虽然柔细，但再结实的土也不能阻挡，所以说木能疏土，即木能克土；土能阻水，土堤能防水之流溢、泛滥，且水坑填土后，坑平而水干，故土能克水；水能灭火，所以水能克火；火能溶化金属，所以火能克金；金属刀具能伐木，故金能克木。所以《素问·宝命全形论》说："木得金而伐，火得水而灭，土得木而达，金得火而缺，水得土而绝。"

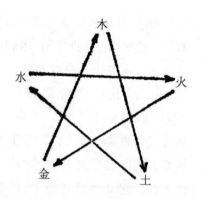

图9　五行相克图

《内经》把五行"相克"关系称为"承制"关系，承是承袭的意思，制是监制的意思。承制，即后者对前者承袭而监制之意。如《素问·六微旨大论》说："相火之下，水气承之；水位之下，土气承之。"水在相火之下，既承袭相火之气，又对相火发生监制作用；土在水位之下，既承袭了水气，同时又有监制水气的作用。《内经》又把五行"相克"关系称为"相胜"关系，即相加后必然能胜的意思。又把被我所"克"者称为"所胜"，即我所能胜；把"克"我者称为"所不胜"，即我所不能胜。以木为例，金克木，故木不能胜金，金为木之"所不胜"；木克土，故木能胜土，土为木之"所胜"。

在五行的相互关系中，每一行都要和其他四行发生联系。这种联系不外是"相生"和"相克"，其"相生"的关系有二，即一为"生我"，一为"我生"；"相克"的关系也有二，即一为"克我"，一为"我克"。以木为例，木和水、火二行是"相生"的关系，水生木，木生火，故对木而言，水为木之"生我"，火为木之"我生"；木和金，土二行是"相克"的关系，金克木、木克土，故对木而言，金为木之"克我"，土为木之"我克"。五行之中的每一"行"都要通过"生""克"的方式而和其他四"行"发生联系，它既要受到其他"行"的制约，它又要对其他"行"发生制约作用。这样就在五行间形成了相互依存又相互制约的关系，从而维持了它们之间的相互平衡和协调，使五行成

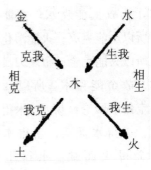

图 10 木和其他四行的生克关系图

为一个有机的整体。于是，五行中的每一"行"都不能脱离其他四"行"而单独存在，任何一"行"的变化，都要对其他四"行"发生影响，也要受到其他四"行"对它的作用。正因为这个原因，五行就成为一个相当严密而又相当稳定的结构。

（2）五行的乘侮　五行"乘侮"是五行间的异常联系方式，它是由于五行间"量"的异常而引起的克制异常或克制太过的现象。

"乘"，又称"相乘"，是乘袭的意思，即乘虚而袭之，是克制太过的表现。"侮"，又称为"相侮"，"反侮"，是恃己之强，凌彼之弱，侮所不胜的现象，"相侮"也是一种克制的异常，主要表现为反向克制，即与正常相克的方向相反，所以又称"反克"。

五行"乘侮"发生的原因有二：一是由于该"行"太过，

超出了五行间平衡所允许的波动范围，出现了异常的过盛。异常过盛的结果，必然对它所克制的一"行"（即所胜）进行过度的克制，即"相乘"；同时也对克制它的一"行"（即所不胜）进行"反克"，即"相侮"。二是由于该"行"过度衰弱，超出了五行间平衡所允许的波动范围，出现了异常的不足。异常的不足，使该"行"对其所克制的一"行"（所胜）

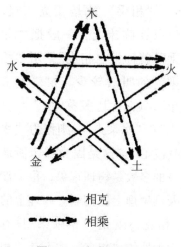

图11　五行相乘图

无力克制，反而对它进行"反克"，即"相侮"；克制它的一"行"（所不胜），则因它的异常不足，出现了相对的克制过甚，即"相乘"。《素问·五运行大论》说："气有余，则制己所胜，而侮所不胜；其不及，则己所不胜，侮而乘之，己所胜，轻而侮之。"就是说的这个意思。五行"相乘"是克制超过了正常范围的克制太过的现象，它在克制的方向上并没有异常，所以，五行"相乘"的方向和五行"相克"的方向是一致的，也是木乘土、土乘水、水乘火、火乘金、金乘木。

五行"相侮"是由于五行盛衰超出了正常允许的范围，而引起的一种异常克制。它可能在克制的强度上有所异常，但主要的是在克制的方向上，出现了反向的克制。即和五行正常克制的方向相反，所以又称"反克"。五行"相侮"的顺序是：木侮金、金侮火、火侮水、水侮土，土侮木。

"相乘"就是相克太过，所以在临床上，一般把"相乘"就称为"相克"，用"相乘"的叫法较少。如"木乘土"，临床上多称为"木克土"；"水乘火"，则称为"水气凌心"。这是因为临床所涉及的多数是病理现象，很少涉及到生理上的克制。病理上的"相克"就是"相乘"，只有生理性的"相克"才不是"相乘"。

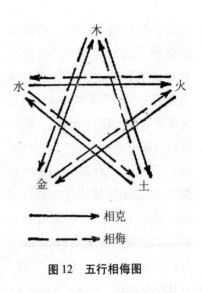

图12 五行相侮图

"相侮"在临床上的称法很不统一，如"土侮木"，即称为"土壅木郁"；"木侮金"即称为"木火刑金"；其他如"心火下灼肾阴"即是"火侮水"的现象，"肺热传心"即是"金侮火"的病理表现。

（3）五行的生克制化 五行之间存在着"相生"和"相克"这两种联系方式，它维持了事物内部的平衡和协调关系，也就维护了事物的稳定性、统一性和整体性，维护了事物正常的运动变化，即维护了事物正常的生命过程。"制"即监制、制约，即起到控制作用；事物内部各构成部分之间的相互监制、制约，维持了它们之间的平衡和协调，因而也就维护了事物的稳定性、统一性和整体性。"化"即变化，是指事物在内部统一、协调和平衡的状态下而发生的正常运动变化。

《素问·六微旨大论》说："亢则害，承乃制，制则生化，外列盛衰，害则败乱，生化大病。"如果五行之中的某一"行"出现了亢盛的现象，就要引起五行间关系的失常（即"害"）；如果五行之间相互承袭，五行之间就有正常的监制或制约作用，五行间的关系就正常。五行间有正常的相互监制或制约作用，就维护了五行之间的平衡和协调，事物就能发生正常的生长变化，在外面就表现出来有盛有衰的正常生命过程；五行间相互关系失去了正常，不能发挥正常的监制或制约作用，事物内部的平衡和协调关系就要被破坏，而发生紊乱（败乱），正常的生长变化运动就不能维持。这说明了，严重的"生化"紊乱就要威胁到事物的生命及其存在（发生大病）。《内经》认为，五行间的"生克制化"维护了事物的存在和正常的生命活动。

明·张景岳所著的《类经图翼》说："盖造化之机，不可无生，亦不可无制，无生则发育无由，无制则亢而为害。"世界上万物的产生和运动变化的微妙之处是：既不可以没有相互资生的作用，也不可以没有相互监制或制约的作用。如果没有相互资生的作用，那么事物的产生和生长变化就没有来源了；如果没有相互监制或制约的作用，事物内部各构成部分之间就要出现偏亢偏衰的现象，它们之间的平衡和协调关系就要被破坏，事物的正常生命过程或事物的存在就要受到威胁。所以，张景岳也认为：五行之间的"生克制化"是维护事物的存在及其生命发生发展过程的根本原因。

关于五行"生克制化"的具体方式，《素问·至真要大论》说："胜至则复，复已则胜，不复则害。"当事物间相克制的力量达到极点（即"胜至"）的时候，就要向它的反面转化（即"复"），出现克制的衰减；当克制衰减到极限（即"复已"）的时候，又要向克制增强（即"胜"）的方向转化。如果没有这种盛衰交替的变化，就要导致事物间正常关系的破坏，危及事物的存在。《素问·天元纪大论》说："形有盛衰，谓五行之治，各有太过不及也。故其始也，有余而往，不足随之；不足而往，有余从之。"事物表现出有盛有衰的过程，是五行间协调节制的结果，各行都有太过和不及的过程，所以，它在开始的时候，随着有余的过去，跟随而来的是不足；随着不足的过去，随之而来的是有余，这是说在事物的存在和发生发展过程中，总表现为盛衰的交替，这是五行调节作用的结果。这说明任何事物或现象的存在和发生发展过程，不是静止的，也不是均衡的，总是在不均衡之中、运动之中来求得均衡，求得平衡和协调，以求得生存和发生发展。这是一个动态过程，是在动态过程中求得平衡和协调，以维护它的稳定性，维护它的存在。

　　在五行之间的相互关系中，也不例外，也是在不均衡中、动态的过程中来求得平衡和协调，以维护五行的统一性、整体性和稳定性。五行之中的各"行"也有自己的盛衰变化，各"行"的盛衰变化，必然要引起该"行""相生"和"相克"发生相应的变化。五行之间"相生"和"相克"作用的目的是维持五行之间的平衡和协调。因而，在正常情况下，五行间"相生"作用的强弱和该"行"的盛衰成正比，五行间"相克"作用的强弱和该"行"的盛衰成反比。即某"行"自身增强时，它"相生"作用也随之而增强，它"相克"作用则随之减弱；反之，如该"行"减弱了，则它"相生"作用也随之减弱，而它"相克"作用却反而增强了。五行自身盛衰和它"相生""相克"作用之间存在这样一种相应的关系，不仅是维护它自身的存在，更重要的是维护五行间的平衡和协调，维护五行的统一性、整体性和稳定性，维护整体存在所必需的。例如在动物界中，缺乏防卫能力的食草类动物，一般具有较强的繁殖能力，过着大群体生活，由数十至数百只组成一群，共同生活在一起；具有进攻能力的猛兽，一般繁殖能力较差，过着小群体生活，由数只至十数只生活在一起。食草动物以它较强的繁殖能力，保证了数量的优势，既满足了食肉动物的食物需要（"相生"作用），又保证了种族的繁衍；食肉动物的繁殖能力虽然差，在数量上处于劣势，但它有强大的进攻和捕获能力（"相克"作用），能获得足够的食物，也保证了它种族的繁衍。食草动物以数量上的优势（自身强盛），保证了对食肉动物的食物供应（"相生"作用强），但却缺乏对攻击者的防卫能力（"相克"作用弱）；食肉动物在数量上的劣势（自身衰弱），决定它对其他生物支持能力不足（"相生"作用弱），而它却有强大的进攻及防卫能力（"相克"作用强）。食草动物、食肉动物以及和其他生物，它们在自身数量对其他生物的支持和自身防卫能力等方面的差异，有助于其本身的生存、种族的繁衍和生态平衡的维持，是自然界繁荣的保证，这都是自然选择的结果。

当五行"相克"作用的强弱和该"行"的盛衰成正比时，它必然导致盛者益盛，衰者益衰，终于引起五行间的平衡和协调关系的破坏，使五行的统一性、整体性和稳定性不能存在，作为一个整体的事物也就不能再继续存在，所以，五行"相克"作用强弱和该"行"的盛衰成正比时，就成为一种破坏因素，是属于五行"相克"的异常状态。

为了说明五行是怎样通过"生克"来维护其平衡和协调，

张景岳提出了五行"生克制化"的具体方式，即五行的"胜复"。《类经图翼》说："自其胜复者盲，则凡有所胜，必有所败；有所败，必有所复；母之败也，子必救之。如水之太过，火受伤矣，火之子土，出而制焉。"从五行的"胜复"来说，凡是有获胜的，必然就有失败的；有了失败的，必然就有为失败进行报复的；"母"败之后，其"子"必然要去援救，如果"水"气太过，"火"气必然要受伤，"火"的"子""土"气，也就出来以制止"水"气。在张氏所举的这个例子中，由于"水"气过盛，超过了正常的范围，出现了异常的克制（克制的力量和该"行"的盛衰成正比）。"水"对"火"的过分克制，引起"火"气的损伤，"火"气受损，则不能"生子"，引起"火"之"子"——"土"气也衰。在正常情况下，五行"相克"力量的强弱，和该"行"的盛衰成反比，所以"土"气增强了对"水"气的克制，使"水"气恢复正常，"水"对"火"的克制力量减弱，"火"气得到复原，"火"生"土"的作用增强，"土"气也就复原，"土"克"水"的力量也随之减弱，三者之间也就恢复了正常的状态。

在上述例子中，"水"对"火"的克制，是属于异常的即病理性克制，所以，"水"克"火"的力量与"水"的盛衰成正比；而"土"对"水"的克制，是属于正常的即生理性的克制，所以，"土"克"水"的力量和"土"的盛衰成反比。这两个克制是不同的。

在上面的例子中，张氏只提到"水""火""土"三者的关系，而未提到"金"和"木"的作用，其实"金"和"木"也参与其中的调节作用。"水"气盛，则"水"生"木"的作用增强；"木"气旺，"木"生"火"的作用也增强，有助于抵制"水"对"火"的克制，防止"火"气过衰；"木"气旺，"木"克"土"的作用减弱，防止了"土"气过衰。"火"被"水"克而衰，则"火"克"金"的作用增强；"火"衰不能生"土"，"土"衰不能生"金"。这都是为了使"金"气变衰，使"金"不能生"水"，以削弱"水"气。所以，在上面的例子中，除了"水""火""土"三者之间发

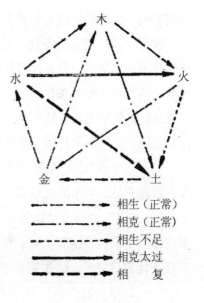

图13　五行胜复图

生的相应的"生克"变化外，"木"和"金"也发生了相应的"生克"变化。一切变化的中心都是为了防止"火""土"二气过衰，遏制"水"气的太过，以使五行之间已经失去的平衡和协调关系，能够迅速地重新建立起来。

五行就是通过"生克制化"以维护其平衡和协调，维护了五行的统一性、整体性和稳定性，也就维护了事物的存在。

（4）五行生克的辩证关系　五行生克的辩证关系，主要表现有两方面：一是五行生克和"量"的关系；二是五行生克的"互用"关系，即"生中有克""克中有用"。

五行生克和"量"的关系，是说五行的生克和五行的"量"（即五行的盛衰）有关，主要是和五行中各"行"的"量"的

比例有关。以上所谈的五行生克规律，仅是就一般"常量"而言，即各"行"盛衰的变化，是限制在五行间平衡和协调所允许的波动范围之内。只有在这种条件下，以上所介绍的五行生克规律才能成立。如果条件发生了变化，当五行间盛衰的变化超过了所允许的波动范围，特别是五行间盛衰的比例超出了所允许的波动范围，上述的五行生克规律也就不能成立了。

如"水生木"，这是就"水"和"木"盛衰的比例相当而言，水源充足，草木的生长就旺盛。如"水"和"木"的比例不相当，"水"少则不足以解救已成之旱，虽然有"水"，但草木也难以生长；"水"太过，泛滥成灾，其不仅不能生"木"，而且还能害"木"，已生成的草木反能被成灾之水淹没而死。"木生火"，也是就"木"和"火"盛衰的比例相当而言。如在小堆之火中投以巨木，则火不仅不能焰，反而被巨木所压灭。所以，"母"和"子""量"的关系必须相当，即"母""子"双方的"量"只能限制在平衡允许的波动范围之内，才有上述的"相生"关系；如双方"量"的比例不能相当，超出了平衡允许的波动范围，则"母"生"子"的关系就要被破坏，即"壮母"不能生"弱子"，或"弱母"不能生"壮子"。

五行"相克"的关系也只能限制在常量的范围之内，如超出了平衡允许的波动范围，上述的"相克"规律也不能成立。"土克水"，只有在二者比例相当的条件下，土堤才能防止洪水的泛滥，如山洪暴发，洪水倾泻，一般的土堤不仅不能防止，反而会被山洪冲垮，而无制"水"的作用。"水克火"，但用一杯水去救熊熊的烈火，这水不但不能灭火，反能助火之炎。这说明在"相克"的过程中，克制和被克制双方在"量"的比例上，也必须相当。双方比例不相当，它们的克制关系也随之改变。

所以说，在五行生克的关系中，都存在着"量"的关系。只有在"生克"双方在"量"的比例相当时，五行的"生克"才有一定的顺序；五行间"量"的比例不相当时，"五行倒转相克"其意思也就是在于此。

五行"生克"只有在"常量"的范围，其顺序才能成立，这是说五行之间盛衰的比例关系。这种比例关系，实际上是说五行的盛衰波动，只能限制在五行间平衡和协调所允许的波动范围之内，这是属于正常的波动，超出这个波动范围，则属异常现象，必然要引起异常的克制，即属于五行的"乘侮"关系。

五行的生克"互用"，即张景岳所说的"生中有克""克中有用"。《类经图翼》说："第人知夫生之为生，而不知生中有克；知克之为克，而不知克中有用。"一般人只知道五行的"相生"就是相互资生，而不知道在相互资生中包含着相互克制；只知道五行的"相克"就是相互克制，而不知道相互克制的目的是发挥被克制者的正常作用。张景岳认识到"相生"中存在着"相克"和"相残"的作用，而"相克"的目的是"克以致用"，即包含有"相生"和"互用"的意思。如"木生火"，"木"被"火"焚而化为灰烬，"木"已不复存在；"火生土"，物被"火"焚而成灰，灰即是"土"，灰积太多，"火"被灰伏而不能炎。"木"使"火"旺，"火"旺则"木"反受其害；"火"使"土"增，"土"增则反而伏"火"。五行"相生"的结果是"子"成而"母"被"子"害。所以说，五行的"相生"中包含有"相克"或"相残"的意思，即出现"子"克"母"或"子"害"母"的现象。

五行"相克"是为了发挥被克者的正常功能，如"水克火"，"火"被"水"克而成"水火既济"，使"火"不过于炽盛，而能发挥"火"温煦功能。如"水"不制"火"，"火"盛必成燎原之势，焚毁万物，反而成灾。"土克水"，"水"被"土"克，使"水"气受制，而不至于太过，则能发挥"水"的滋润、济火的功能。如"土"不制"水"，"水"气无制，必然流溢为害，泛滥成灾。所以说，五行"相克"的目的是为了对被克制者进行控制，以使它发挥正常的功能，即"克以致用"。

以上说明了五行"相生"的实质是"转化"，即由"母"转化为"子"；五行"相克"的实质是为了使被克制者发挥正常的功能，即包含有"相生""互用"的含义。"相生"和"相克"是相反相成的关系，是辩证的关系。

（三）五行学说在医学上的应用

1. 表达了人与自然的统一性

五行学说把人体的结构与功能分属于五行，又将自然界的五季、五方、五时、五气、五味、五色等也分属于五行，通过五行把自然界和人体统一起来，成为一个整体。使"天人一体""天人相应"的理论得到了具体的表达，为中医学的整体观念提供了理论根据。

人体与自然界统一简表

自然界							五 行 及其属性	人 体					
五色	五味	五气	五时	五化	五方	五季		五脏	五腑	五体	五官	五神	五志
青	酸	风	平旦	生	东	春	木（生发舒展）	肝	胆	筋	目	魂	怒
赤	苦	暑	日中	长	南	夏	火（温热炎上）	心	小肠	脉	舌	神	喜
黄	甘	温	日西	化	中	长夏	土（长养变化）	脾	胃	肉	口	意	思
白	辛	燥	合夜	收	西	秋	金（清肃收敛）	肺	大肠	皮毛	鼻	魄	悲
黑	咸	寒	夜半	藏	北	冬	水（寒湿下行）	肾	膀胱	骨	耳	志	恐

通过五行的联系，人体和自然界统一起来，如五脏和季节的关系是：肝气旺于春，心气旺于夏，脾气旺于长夏，肺气旺于秋，肾气旺于冬，肝病畏秋季，心病畏冬季，脾病畏春季，肺病畏夏季，肾病畏长夏。五脏和五气的关系是：风伤肝，暑伤心，湿伤脾，燥伤肺，寒伤肾。自然界的各种现象都可以通过这种关系和人体联系起来，说明"天人相应"的具体内容。

2. 建立了人体生理学理论

（1）以五行属性阐明五脏生理功能　五行学说将五脏归属于五行，并以五行的属性来阐明五脏的生理功能。木性曲直，性喜舒展，有生发的特性；肝与木气相通，故肝喜条达，主疏泄，主升。火性温热，其性炎上；心与火气相通，故主温煦，主血脉之运行，而温养全身。土性敦厚，生化万物，主长养变化；脾与土气相通，主运化水谷精微，为后天之本，生化之源。金性清凉洁净，主肃降收敛，肺通金气，主呼吸，司清浊之交换，其气主降。水性寒湿润下，而主闭藏，肾通水气，故主封藏，藏精而掌水液之气化。以五行的属性，说明五脏生理特性，是五行学说在医学上运用的一个重要方面。

五行属性和五脏生理功能简表

五行	五行属性	五脏	五脏生理
木	曲直、生发、舒展	肝	喜条达、主疏泄、主升
火	温热、炎上	心	主温煦、主血脉、温养全身
土	长养变化	脾	运化水谷精微、为生化之源
金	清肃收敛	肺	主呼吸清浊、肃降而行水
水	寒湿、润下、闭藏	肾	主封藏、藏精、纳气、水液气化

（2）以五行生克制化阐明五脏的生理联系　五行学说以五行生克制化的理论，阐明五脏之间的生理联系，从而把五脏组合成一个有机的整体。用五脏之间的互助和制约来说明维护人体内部平衡和协调的机理，为证明人是一个有机的整体提供了理论依据。

以五行"相生"说明五脏间的互助关系：

木生火：肝血濡养心神。

火生土：心阳温运脾阳。（《内经》以"心火"为人身阳气之源立论，后世则以"肾火"为人身阳气之根本，故后多以"肾阳温运脾阳"。）

土生金：脾气散精，上归于肺，以养肺气。

金生水：肺气肃降，通调水道，以助肾气行水。

水生木：肾阴滋养肝阴，即水能涵木。

以五行"相克"说明五脏间的制约关系：

木克土：肝气条达，以疏泄脾气，使脾气能够运化。

水克火：肾水上济于心，以制止心火上炎，而成水火既济。

土克水：脾气运化，以助肾气行水。

火克金：心阳温煦，以制肺金清肃太过。

金克木：肺气肃降，以制肝气升发过度。

五脏间的相助和相制，维护了五脏间处于平衡和协调状态，维护了人体生命功能的正常。

（3）建立人体生理系统五行学说 把人体组织、结构、脏腑、器官，以及生理功能和生命现象，都归属于五行，形成了以五脏为中心的五个生理系统。又以五行间的相互关系来说明五脏之间的功能联系，以五脏来统一人体，使人体成为一个有机的整体。

人体生理系统简表

五行	五脏	六腑	形体	五官九窍	五神	五志	五液	五荣	五脉
木	肝	胆	筋	目	魂	怒	泪	爪	弦
火	心	小肠	脉	舌	神	喜	汗	面色	洪
土	脾	胃	肌肉	口	意	思	涎	唇	缓
金	肺	大肠	皮毛	鼻	魄	悲忧	涕	毛	浮
水	肾	膀胱三焦	骨	耳、二阴	志	恐	唾	发	沉

以五行学说为基础建立起来的人体生理系统，是以五脏为核心，各系统的各构成部分都在该脏的统率下，进行自己的生理活

动。如六腑、形体、五官（九窍）、五液、五荣等功能均有赖于五脏，如胆要赖肝气疏泄，小肠要赖心阳的温煦，胃要赖脾气升清，大肠要赖肺气肃降，膀胱和三焦要赖肾气的蒸化等；有的本身就是五脏生理功能的表现，如五神、五志、五荣、五脉等。

以五行学说为基础建立起来的人体生理系统，更进一步确立了人是一个完整有机整体的基本概念。

3. 建立了病理学理论

（1）病因学理论　根据五行学说建立起来的人体与自然的统一关系，提出了风气入肝、火（暑）气入心、湿气入脾、燥气入肺、寒气入肾的理论。同理又推出肝病易见动风，心病易见火热，脾病易见湿阻，肺病易伤津化燥，肾病易从寒化。

（2）建立五脏病的传变理论　根据五行生克制化的关系，提出五脏病的传变理论。五脏病的传变可沿"相生"或"相克"途径传变。沿"相生"的途径传变，病由母脏传及子脏，称为"母病及子"。如肾为水脏，肝为木脏，水能生木，故肾为母脏，肝为子脏。如病先有肾精不足，进之引起肝血亏损，导致肝肾精血俱亏；或是先有肾水亏损，不能滋养肝木，而成肝肾阴虚，肝阳上亢，又称"水不涵木"。凡此种种皆属"母病及子"。《难经》把"母病及子"的传变方式称为"间传"，并提出"间传则生"，认为按此方式传变的疾病，预后良好。

如病由子脏而传及母脏的称为"子盗母气"。心为火脏，肝为木脏，木能主火，故肝为母脏，心为子脏。如先有劳神过度，暗耗心血，累及于肝，致肝血亏损，而成心肝血虚；或先有心火上炎，累及于肝，一而致心肝火旺。此皆属子病累母，"子盗母气"。

病变如沿"相克"的途径传变，即称"相乘"。如因情志不舒，肝气失于条达，而致肝气郁结，横逆犯于脾土，致脾失运化，此即肝气犯脾，又称"木克土"。先有脾气虚弱，久之脾阳也虚，下及肾阳，导致脾肾阳虚；先有心火上炎，日久耗及肺阴，而成心肺阴虚火旺之证。此等皆沿"相克"方向传变，谓之"相乘"，《难经》称为"七传"，并提出"七传则死"，认为按此途径传变者，预后不佳。

病变如逆"相克"方向传变的，称为"相侮"或"反侮"，又称"反克"。如先有食伤而致脾气壅滞，累及于肝，使肝气失于条达，即成"土壅木郁"之证。如先有心阳不足，下吸肾阳，致肾阳也虚，不能制水，终成阴寒极盛之"水气凌心"之证。先有肝火偏亢，阴液暗耗，久之累及于肺，更伤肺阴，成"木火刑金"之证。此等皆属"相侮"之证。

用五行生克的理论来认识五脏疾病的传变，是有一定的临床意义的。临床上常见的如肝气犯胃、肝气犯脾、木火刑金、水气凌心、水气射肺、土壅木郁、心脾两虚、脾肾两虚、肝肾阴虚、心肾不交诸证都和五行生克有一定关系。但是，疾病的传变是复杂的，如《素问·玉机真脏论》说："然其卒发者，不必治于传，或其传化有不以次。"然而，如是突发病，就不必按五行生克关系去先治其应传变的脏腑，或者它的传变也有不是按照五行生克顺序进行的。这说明了，按五行生克来认识五脏疾病的传变，虽有一定的价值，但也不是唯一的传变规律，当灵活地看待。

4. 为中医诊断学提供了理论根据

《灵枢·本脏》说："视其外应，以知其内脏，则知所病矣。"察看内脏在体表相应部位，可以用此来推测内脏情况，这就可以知道它所患的疾病。人是一个有机的整体，内脏有病必然会反映到体表，即"有诸内者，必形诸外"。

内脏有病时，引起内脏生理功能及与其相关内脏的相互关系发生变化，可以反映到体表，而引起色泽、声音、形态、味觉、脉象等的变化。《难经》说："望而知之者，望见其五色，以治其病；闻而知之者，闻其五音，以别其病；问而知之者，问其所欲五味，以知其病所起所在也；切脉而知之者，诊其寸口，视其虚实，以知其病，病在何脏腑也。"通过望的方法而知道病情的人，就是望他的五色的变化，根据色泽变化来了解病情。通过听的方法而知道病情的人，就是听他五音的变化，来辨别病情。通过询问的方法来诊断疾病的人，是问病人对五味的好恶，从而知道疾病是怎样发生的，病变在什么部位。通过切脉的方法而诊断疾病的人，就是诊他寸口脉，辨它的虚实，从而知道他的病情，其病在什么脏腑。这里提出中医诊断疾病的基本方法是望、闻、问、切四法，即称"四诊"。

对"四诊"方法所取的临床症状，按五行学说的理论，分别归属五脏，从而判断病变的部位和程度，以作出诊断。这就是根据五行学说把临床表现在色泽、味觉、脉象等方面的变化，分属五脏，作为诊断的依据。

五脏病变简表

五行	五脏病	五劳	五色	五味	形体	五官	脉象	症状
木	肝病	久行伤筋	青	酸	筋急	目糊	弦	胁支满
火	心病	久视伤血	赤	苦	脉阻	舌赤	洪	心烦神乱
土	脾病	久坐伤肉	黄	甘	肉削	口腻	濡缓	腹胀食少
金	肺病	久卧伤气	白	辛	毛焦	鼻塞	浮	咳喘气短
水	肾病	久立伤骨	黑	咸	骨萎	耳聋	沉	厥，腰痛腿软

如见面青、嗜酸、脉弦等为肝病；面赤、口苦、脉洪等为心病。这是根据症状的表现和脏腑的关系，来判断疾病的部位。

如所患为脾胃病，其面色当黄，脉象当濡缓，反见面色发青，或脉弦，为肝来犯脾。如所患为心脏病，其面色当红，脉象当洪数，反见面色暗黑，脉象沉微细数，为水克火的征象，为"水气凌心"。这是根据病变中出现临床症状有不一致的征象，来判断病情的转变和疾病中脏腑间的相互关系。

5. 建立了中医治疗学理论

在临床治疗时，也要根据五行生克制化的理论，来调整脏腑的功能及其相互关系。

《难经》说："见肝之病，则知肝当传之于脾，故当先实其脾。"当看到肝病时，由于肝能克脾（木克土），所以知道肝病最易传脾，应当先充实脾气，使肝病不至于传脾。这就是《内经》"先安未受邪之地"的"治未病"思想的具体运用。

对虚证和实证的治疗，也可根据五行生克制化的理论来进行调整。根据"母能养子"和"子赖母气"的关系，对虚、实证治疗的基本原则是"虚则补其母""实则泻其子"，对于虚证，可以通过补其母脏来达到补其病脏的目的；对于实证，可以通过泻其子脏来达到泻其病脏的目的。"培土生金"是治肺脏虚证的常用方法，根据"土生金"的关系，补益脾气就能起到补肺的目的，这就是"虚则补其母"的方法。在肝火亢盛的情况下，由于火为木子，所以可以用泻心火的方法达到泻肝火的目的，这就是"实则泻其子"方法。

运用五行相生的原理提出的治疗法则，如滋水涵木法、益火补土法、培土生金法、金水相生法等；根据五行相克的原理提出的治疗法则，如扶土抑木法、培土制水法、佐金平木法、泻南补北法等。

在针灸治疗时，也同样可以使用这些原理进行指导。

6. 在中药学理论方面的运用

五行学说在中药学理论方面的运用，主要是从五味上来概括药物的作用以及它和五脏的关系。

五味，即是指药物的气味，可分酸、苦、甘、辛、咸五味。五味的作用各不相同，《素问·脏气法时论》说："辛散，酸收，甘缓，苦坚，咸软。"辛味药有发散的作用，多用于发散风寒或疏利气机；酸味药有收敛止涩，生津止渴的作用，可用于收敛津气，固肠止泻以及津伤口渴之时；甘味药有缓和止痛、补益的作用，可用于治疗虚证，脾胃不和，拘急疼痛。苦味药有坚阴、泻火、燥湿、通泄的作用，可用于肾气不坚。火毒炽盛，湿热并重，腑气不通之时；咸味药软坚散结，润燥救液，可用于癥瘕积聚，肿块不消，阴液亏损之时。五味，是选用药物的根据之一。

根据五行学说的理论，五味还和五脏相关。《素问·至真要大论》说："酸先入肝，苦先入心，甘先入脾，辛先入肺，咸先入肾。"说明五味入口后，各有所归。另一方面，正因为五味各有所归，所以，它既可补脏，也可伤脏，如酸味药能补肝，但用之过度，反能伤肝。

（四）阴阳学说和五行学说

阴阳学说和五行学说原是我国古代两种哲学理论，在战国末期融合而为阴阳五行学说。中医学理论引进的主要是融合后的阴阳五行学说。

阴阳学说和五行学说已分别介绍于前，都是我国古代朴素的唯物论和辩证法思想，两种学说既有相同的一面，也有不同的一面。

1. 阴阳学说和五行学说的共同点

（1）二者都是我国古代朴素的唯物论和辩证法思想。

（2）二者都是研究一个相对独立的整体及其内部稳定性的维持方式和方法。

（3）二者都采用类比的方法来对事物或现象进行归类，用"同构"的理论进行认识。

（4）二者都建立在"平衡论"的基础上，都以"平衡"和"协调"来说明事物的稳定状态，以"互生"和"互制"两种方式来说明事物间的联系方式，并以这两种联系方式构成的"自调系统"来维持事物内部的"平衡"和"协调"，以及事物的运动、发展和变化。

（5）"阴阳"和"五行"都是抽象的、相对的概念，都不是指特定的事物或现象，但在属性上都具有规定性。

（6）二者都以超越正常的"生""制"作用作为异常或病理现象。

2. 阴阳学说和五行学说的相互补充

（1）阴阳学说以"二"为基数。在数学上是"二进位制"，在方法论上是"二分法"。五行学说是以"五"为基数，在数学上是"十进位制"，在方法论上是"多分法"。

（2）在维持事物内部平衡和协调（即自动调节）的方式上，阴阳学说是采用"直接负反馈"的方式，五行学说是采用"间接负反馈"方式。

（3）阴阳五行学说是采用阴阳之中分五行、五行之中分阴阳的方法，把两种理论融合为一体，合并应用。在中医学理论中，分析生理或病理现象时，既分五脏，又分阴阳，在五脏之中分阴阳（如每个脏腑均有阴阳、气血），阴阳之中分五脏（如人体分阴阳，阴中有五脏，阳中有五腑）。

Foreword

Traditional Chinese Medicine(referred to as "TCM") is a science with long history, unique theoretical system and rich clinical experience. It glitters with growing splendor in medicine all over the world. International and domestic scholars find immense stock of TCM and its profound influence to world science. Thus, it is very popular to study TCM and Chinese culture now.

Yin-yang and five elements theory is a important theoretical basis of TCM and the core factor constructed through the formation of the world outlook and methodology of TCM. It is also where both holism and view of nature are rooted. However, the theory is relatively abstract, profound and extensive in the scope of statements, and archaic and abstruse in logic and grammar, so it is hard to understand, especially for beginners. For this reason, Zhu Zongyuan wrote Yin-yang and Five-element Theory in 1987. The book details the basic connotation of yin-yang and five-element theory, including the nature of TCM, formation of TCM theoretical system, yin-yang theory, five-element theory and so on. It provides a reference of learning the theory for beginners and TCM amateurs.

Professor Zhu, of Inner Mongolia Medical University, has been teaching and studying basic theories of TCM for several decades. He

101

studies classic medical works and never rigidly adheres to them but chooses and follows what are right. In the researches and inheritance of TCM theory and culture, he strives for increasing perfection and has his own original understanding. Prof. Zhu always says that if TCM theory is able to spread at home and abroad, it will contribute more for the development of TCM science.

Based on the inexorable trend and urgent demands of human bioscience, with Mr. Zhu's support and guidance and the purpose of fulfilling his wish, We revises and translates Yin-yang and Five Elements Theory into English, and issues at home and abroad, expect to improve the academic communication of TCM.

The book incorporates abundant data, explains the profound with simple terms, and includes detailed illustrations. The author expects that it is able to open a way for medical science so as to function better for the development of TCM.

Yang Guoying

Introduction

Traditional Chinese medicine (TCM) has a history of thousands of years, and it is one of the most ancient medical schools that existing. It is the result of Chinese people's long-term fight with diseases, a precious cultural legacy of Chinese nation, and embodying oriental civilization. During the formation of the TCM theoretical system, it took in the thoughts of the ancient materialism and dialectics as its own guiding ideology and methodology, and gradually developed a set of unique theoretical system of medicine, standing tall worldwide and contributing a lot for the national health and prosperity. Until today, TCM theory still has scientific values, and it attracts much attention in the global medical field. This is the reason why we still study and carry forward it with the hope that it will play an important role in the development of human health and life sciences in the near future.

Part I What is TCM

Almost everyone has heard of the name—TCM, but it is another thing to know it. TCM actually has two meanings, the generalized one and the narrow-sensed one.

In ancient China, there was only one kind of medicine, without the name—TCM then. With the introduction of the western medicine, the name "foreign medicine" came into being. Especially after the O-pium War, the western medicine poured into China, leading to the co-existence of the two medicines. In order to distinguish them, the national medicine came up as a correspondence to the western medicine. The former is the traditional medicine specific to China, and the latter is the medicine introduced from the western countries. From a-bout 40 to 50 years ago, the "foreign medicine" evolved into "western medicine", and the "national medicine" into TCM. This is the origin of TCM.

Since TCM is specific to China, it should contain all kinds of traditional medicines originated from here, which is what TCM generally implies.

China is a multi-ethnic country, so the traditional medicines originated from here are plenty, such as Tibetan medicine from areas inhabited by Tibetans, Mongolian medicine from areas inhabited by

104

Mongolians, as well as others like Uighur medicine, Miao medicine, Dai medicine, and so on. They are different from the Han medicine originated from areas inhabited by the Han people. Even herbal medicine and snake medicine originated from Han area are quite different from Han medicine. Therefore, the generalized TCM should include all medicine originated from China, such as Han medicine, Tibetan medicine, Mongolian medicine, Uighur medicine, Dai medicine, herbal medicine and snake medicine.

In most cases, when we use the word "TCM", it does not include all the traditional medicines of China but only refers to Han medicine. This is due to its large and dense population wide inhabitation in culturally and economically developed places. Han medicine is the most common method for health care. It has the greatest effect at home. It also has a certain effect in the foreign countries. On the other hand, because of the ethnic isolation, other kinds of medicine did not get widely spread and well known to the Han people. Therefore, Han medicine is automatically considered as TCM. Despite the impreciseness, it has been an idiom. This is the second implication of TCM, i. e. the narrow-sensed meaning.

Part II The Nature of TCM

1. TCM is within the scope of traditional medicine

The World Health Organization (WHO) divides the existing medicines into two categories: the modern medicine and the traditional medicine. Based on the western traditional medicine and with the development of modern scientific technology, the modern medicine takes shape in the recent 200 to 300 years. It is the product of the combination of western traditional medicine and modern scientific technology. Since the dependence on experiments, it is also called "experimental medicine". The traditional medicine has a long history. It gradually came into being with the humans' appearance, accumulating a lot of people's experience on long-term fight with diseases. Clinical experience is the source of its development, so it is also called "empirical medicine".

TCM is within the scope of the traditional medicine, and is the biggest medical school with highest development level among the existing traditional medicines, most of which remain at the stage of empirical medicine. For example, in Africa, South Africa and other districts, the traditional medicines are mainly based on rich medical experience. Together with effective drugs, they constitute the major part of the medicine. Despite abundant treatment experience which really is

106

effective for some diseases, they lack complete theories. What's more, as to guiding function in clinical practices, experience is more important than the theories. Nevertheless, TCM is different. Though the clinical experience is its source, it also has a relatively complete theory which plays a more significant role than experience during treatment. It indicates that TCM has risen from the empirical stage to the theoretical one. Therefore, unlike the average traditional medicine, TCM is higher in theoretical level.

2. TCM is a combination of the empirical medicine and the ancient philosophy

There are three reasons that TCM can establish a complete medical theoretical system. One is that it was combined with the Chinese ancient philosophy — the yin-yang and five-element theory at the beginning of its formation, applied the naive materialism and dialectical ideas as guiding ideology and methodology, and organized the medical experience into theories, so as to form a set of unique medical theoretical system. The second one is that governments of the past dynasties took medical science seriously. For example, since the Zhou Dynasty the medical officer system had been set up and divided into several departments, which promoted the medicine to development in depth and breadth. From the Southern and Northern Dynasties, the medical education was established which promoted studies on medical theories. Besides, through all dynasties, it is by governments that forces were assembled to commence the summary and organization of medicine and pharmacy, compile medical formulary and pharmaceutical books of times, which promoted the development of TCM. The third one is that the Chinese nation traditionally attaches importance to medicine. Many ideologists, scientists and militarists join the medical researches, enrich it with knowledge of multiple disciplines, and promote medical theories to develop in depth and breadth and further enhancement and improvement.

Among those reasons above, the combination of medicine and ancient philosophy is the key factor that TCM can achieve high level. The permeation of other disciplines to medicine not only enriches medical theories and constantly integrates the theoretical system, but also ensures the correctness of the guiding ideology from the perspective of epistemology. Thus TCM can set up a high-level and rather perfect theoretical system.

3. The epistemology of TCM

TCM is not based on the empirical medicine. Guided by the idea of similarity between man and nature, through a mass of observation to planets, nature, society and human bodies, with the application of analogy, it learns human bodies and diseases based on natural and social laws and phenomena and treats them in a holistic, dynamic and dialectical way. This method is macrocosmic, intuitional and logical. It studies human bodies through living ones, learns human structure and motion law as well as occurrence and development of diseases in movements, which is obviously different from the epistemic way of modern medicine, even better in some aspects.

Despite the advantages above, there are also some disadvantages. TCM is lack of experimental measures and insufficient in the microcosmic aspect. As a result, the knowledge in human bodies and diseases is not profound enough, and some is even wrong. Besides, the traditional research methods of TCM mainly depend on accumulation of massive clinical materials. They provided abundant medical materials for the formation and development of TCM theories but backward and defective to some extent. To discover problems and summarize laws at the early stage of medical formation were advisable and fruitful. While nowadays when most medical laws have been found, this method will lower the probability of success and prolong the research cycle which may cost dozens of generations to complete the accumulation of experience. It is like finding Yuhua pebbles under the stone piles of Yuhuatai. Before it was well known, people seldom went for it. As long as with patience and diligence, in a half or one day the beautiful ones would always be found. Then with the rising fame of the pebbles, more and more people strive for them whereas less and less pebbles remain. In this situation, much efforts and time are needed even though sometimes there is no result. That is why the research methods of TCM can not meet the needs of the medicine development. In contrast, it becomes the main reason for its slow pace. To change this situation, it is necessary to change the research methods and techniques, shorten the research circle and increase efficiency, so as to accelerate its development.

The other disadvantage is that the TCM research methods are solely based on clinical curative effects. It is unreliable because the curative effects are affected by various factors. A correct treatment is the usual reason for recovery, but there are also many coincident cases of recovery from ineffective treatment. Therefore, it is inappropriate to consider that the doctor's cognition about the disease is right and the therapy is proper just in terms of recovery. Because of this, the TCM theories are inevitably mixed with some unreliable factors.

Every doctor's clinical experience has its one-sidedness, so are the theories derived from it, which is one of the reasons for theoretical divergence. Moreover, they are unrepeatable by the later generations, so they cannot be affirmed or denied. This makes some cases in the TCM theories suspended for a long term, and descendants cannot figure them out. The more cases there are, the more TCM literatures there will be. It is one of reasons that hinder the theoretical development of TCM.

Part Ⅲ The Formation of the TCM Theoretical System

The TCM theoretical system formed during the Qin-Han Dynasty. The forming course lasts thousands of years and can be divided into three stages, i. e. accumulation of medical knowledge, sprout of medical theories and establishment of the TCM theoretical system.

1. The accumulation of medical knowledge

Medicine is formed with the appearance of human beings. The earliest medical activities are actually out of the survival instinct of the primitive men. It was transformed into a kind of knowledge and accumulated as medical experience only after the human intelligence gets evolved by working for the purpose of survival and reproduction. The accumulation of medical experience strengthens humans' understanding of diseases, enriches medical knowledge and becomes the materials of medical theories.

The accumulation of medical knowledge went through a very long time, including the time before the Spring and Autumn Period (700B. C.). There were no literary records about the ancient humans' medical treatments. The descendents wrote them into annals based on tales and passed them down. According to *The Age of Emperors* by Huangfu Mi of the Western Jin Dynasty, Fu Xi Shi—the legendary first ancestor and the initiator of fishing, hunting and herding, created the "Eight Diagrams" to illustrate pathological mechanism and was considered as the founder of the TCM theories. It was said that he created the nine classical needles (including various needles for acupuncture and nine kinds of medical instruments for the incision of abscess). *Wei Li* by people of the Western Han Dynasty recorded the fire discoverers — Suiren Shi drilled wood to make fire, and taught people to eat cooked food to avoid gastrointestinal diseases. According to *Huai Nan Zi* by Liu An who was the king of the Huainan State during the Western Han Dynasty, the creator of agriculture and medicine — Shennong Shi looked for herbal medicine and tasted herbs in person, which sometimes resulted in toxication 70 times a day. In *A-B Classic of Acupuncture and Moxibustion* by Huangfu Mi, it says that in the legend, ruler of the central China — Yellow Emperor, in order to explore the truth of medicine, often talked about human anatomy and physiology with his courtiers Qi Bo, Shao Yu, Bo Gao and so on, and at last illuminated the law of acupuncture. These legends may not be completely true, but the stories reflected Chinese ancient people's contribution to the formation and accumulation of medicine.

It is said that in the Xia Dynasty (the 21st century B. C. – 17th century B. C.), the brewing has been created. *The Strategies of the Warring States* records the story of Yi Di presenting liquor to Xia Yu. The way that doctors treated illnesses with liquor was once a very important treatment, which promoted medical development.

Till the Shang Dynasty (the 16th century B. C. – the 11th century B. C.), medical knowledge got further accumulation, as well as the understanding of diseases. According to the oracle records, during the Wu Ding period, most diseases were recorded generally in terms of pathogenic sites, such as head diseases, eye diseases, ear diseases, abdomen diseases, and so on. It suggests that the division of the human body then was already explicit, while the identification of the symptoms was vague and unspecific. Only a few have particular names, such as malaria, scabies, intoxication, caries, and so on, which indicates that the main features of these diseases had been well understood. People then thought the diseases were out of offence to ancestors, so they mainly prayed or sacrificed for ancestors' forgiveness instead of pursuing treatments. During this time, people also recognized that diseases are relevant to diet, climate and environment, and dancing can strengthen corporeity, prevent and cure some diseases.

In the Western Zhou Dynasty (the 11th century B. C. – 770 B. C.), the medical knowledge was still under slow accumulation, and the awareness of diseases evidently got deepened. Of the 38 diseases recorded in the *Mountain and Sea Classic*, 23 are named according to their major features, such as xia, scabies, wart, subcutaneous ulcer, carbuncle, fistula, heatstroke, goiter, plague, malaria, insanity, hemorrhoids, and so on; 12 of them are named in light of symptoms, such as swelling, deafness, pharyngalgia, cardiodynia, vomit, and so on; only 3 diseases are named by pathogenic sites, like abdomen and heart diseases. Compared with the Wu Ding period, it was an evident progress. Also, 120 kinds of medicinal materials are included

113

in the Mountain and Sea Classic, among which most are vegetal and animal medicine, and the rest are mineral. During this period, though prayer and sacrifice were still the major therapeutic methods, the drug therapy got great development.

Except the progress mentioned above, yin-yang theory and the five-element theory related to TCM were under incubation. The legendary "Eight Diagrams" created by Fu Hsi, through King Wen of Zhou's deduction, became the "Hexagrams", which was an interpretation to the law of opposition and complementarity as well as that of the unity of opposites. During this period, the concepts of "yin-yang" and "five elements" were still in bud. "Yin-yang" was elicited from fronting and backing to the sun. "Five elements" were generalized from the factors indispensable in daily life, and thus it prepared conditions for the formation of "five elements" concept.

2. The embryonic stage of medical theories

The Spring and Autumn Period (770B. C. – 476B. C.) was the time when medical theories formed. One was that ancient philosophical theories as basis of TCM theory formed; the other was that the accumulation of medical knowledge began to transit to theories, and basic viewpoints of TCM took into shape.

The Spring and Autumn Period is also the time when slave society transited to feudal society. Emerging landlord class required a reform and new thoughts were initiated. Hundred schools of thought rose in swarms, and academic atmosphere was unprecedentedly active. Yin-yang theory and five-element theory of naive materialism and dialectical thoughts got a great development. The theoretical system gradually formed and was used to explain various natural and social phenomena.

Yin-yang is formed in the Chinese ancient people's life and labor. It was originally defined in light of fronting and backing to the sun. In *Duan Zhu Shuo Wen*, it says that yin, is south of water and north of mountain; yang is where is high and bright. "It is difficult for sunlight to reach north of mountain and south of water. "Ancient people regarded the places fronting sun or were high as yang side, and those which were lower and can not be shined as yin side. On this basis, yin and yang are taken as symbols of the unity of opposites and abstract concepts with universal meaning instead of specific things or phenomena. According to *Guo Yu*, in the second year of King You of Western Zhou's reign (780 B. C.), there was an earthquake in Sanchuan of Western Zhou. Bo Yang Father thought that when yang-qi is hidden inside and yin-qi is pressed down and cannot vaporize, then earthquake happened. In Zhou Yi, yin-yang is the universe law in nature. It means that yin-yang theory has been in embryo: the first is that yin-yang is law of the nature; the second is that interaction of yin and yang is regarded as the cause of the growth and change of everything in nature; the third is that it helps to establish the concept of yin-yang balance, and the yin-yang disharmony is used to explain abnormal phenomena.

"Five elements", originally called "five materials", was generalized from Chinese people's life and labor. Then they were considered as the basic substances composing all things on earth, meaning "elements" to some extent. Afterwards, the attributes of wood, fire, earth, gold and water were extracted out as abstract concepts illustrating the five elements. Thus, "five elements" became a philosophical concept instead of concrete substances. As an abstract notion, it was thought that the five attributes were contained in all things and phenomena. Therefore, it was introduced in medicine. During this time, the five-element theory was under formation: firstly, "five elements" had been abstracted; secondly, it had been used as natural laws; at last, the main reason that unusual changes occurred was the broken relation of the five elements.

Lao Zi, a famous philosopher at the end of the Spring and Autumn Period, was born about the sixth year of King Jian of Zhou's reign (580 B. C.), and died in the 20th year of King Jing of Zhou's (500 B. C.). He wrote the Lao Zi (also known as Tao Te Ching later) and put forward that firstly the Tao is the core of the world, the source of everything and the harbinger of the essence theory; secondly the idea of "inaction" which means that people should let nature take its course. The theory of "health maintenance" and the idea of "imitating nature" are greatly influenced by Lao Zi. In the book are a lot of dialectics thoughts which exert great influence over TCM theory system.

During the Spring and Autumn Period, the helotism collapsed and the feudal landlord class rose. Especially in the later stage, with the vassal holding more power, the Zhou royalty was weaker, so was theocracy. The aftereffect on medicine was that people began to doubt

116

that ghosts and gods could bring diseases. For example, Zi Chan from Zheng State thought that diseases should be related with daily activities, diet and emotions instead of gods of mountains, rivers or stars. Yan Ying from Qi State also thought that diseases resulted from indulgence in sensual pleasures. According to *Zuo Zhuan*, at the 4th year of King Jing of Zhou's reign (451 B. C.), Yi He from Qin State diagnosed Duke Ping of Jin's disease. He said: "there are six factors in nature. They can generate five flavors, present five colors and produce five tones. Excess of any could bring about six kinds of diseases. The six factors are yin, yang, wind, rain, darkness and brightness. They divide a year into four times and five seasons, and too many divisions will develop into disasters; excessive yin leads to cold diseases; excessive yang leads to fever; excessive wind leads to limb diseases; excessive rain leads to abdomen diseases; excessive darkness leads to mental diseases and excessive brightness leads to heart diseases. " From the statement above, it can be easily inferred that medical theories have been in the embryonic stage at the end of the Spring and Autumn Period and the beginning of the Warring States Period. The basic points of view then are: firstly, the pathogeneses of some diseases were related to nature, society and some other factors and it was believed that undue climates, environment, living habits, emotions and diet, instead of ghosts and gods, could result in diseases; secondly, the idea of "correspondence between man and universe" was introduced into medical theory; thirdly, the concept of "yin-yang" was applied in medicine, proposing that "excessive yin is cold and excessive yang is fever"and Yi which is the origin of what was said in Internal Classic, and the statements about the relation between diseases and wind and rain are also in line with later generations' understanding of wind and damp evils; fourthly, "five elements" was introduced in the medicine, and the concepts of five flavors, five colors and five tones, five seasons and four times, and six factors in nature in fact lay foundation for the related theories in Internal Classic.

After the Spring and Autumn Period, the ancient philosophy referring to medicine achieved a gradual improvement. The accumulation of medical knowledge was on its way to be sublimated as medical theory, which provided sufficient conditions for the formation of TCM theory.

3. The formation of TCM theory

The formation of TCM theory started from the Warring State Period (476B. C. - 221B. C.) and was not completed until the end of the Eastern Han Dynasty (25A. D. - 220A. D.) or the Three Kingdoms Period (220A. D. - 265A. D.). It was marked by the publishment of *Huang Di's Internal Classic*, *Shen Nong's Herbal Classic*, and *Treatise on Febrile and Miscellaneous Diseases*.

(1) The cornerstone of TCM theory——the perfection of the ancient philosophy

To build a house needs a base, which directly affects the quality of the house. TCM theory system has its own foundations, i. e. , abundant treatment experience and medical knowledge. However, after the rise of modern medicine, most traditional medicines are at the edge of extinction except TCM. The key is that at the beginning of its formation, TCM theory system adopted correct ancient philosophy as its own guiding ideology and methodology. It fully utilized ancient philosophical viewpoints and methods, and comprehensively analyzed, deduced and reasoned the abundant treatment experience and medical knowledge, to turn itself into a well-organized, outline-clear, systematic and integrated medical theory system. The ancient philosophical ideologies most closely related to TCM theory are yin-yang theory, five-element theory and essence theory.

Yin-yang theory appeared in the Spring and Autumn Period, and got further development in the Warring States Period. It was widely used because of the abstraction of yin-yang concept. Any thing or phenomenon can be divided into yin and yang parts, i. e. , the original substance forming the universe-essence. The light essences are classified as yang and rise upwards as heaven; the heavy ones are " yin" and fall downwards as earth. What's more, yin-yang's unity of opposites, law of movement, and yin-yang balance are adopted to explain natural and social phenomena. Then yin-yang becomes the fundamental law of movement in nature.

In ancient China, people had learnt the phenomena of being opposite and complementary to each other, and the unity of opposites. The tale "Fu Hsi made Eight Diagrams" was the generalization of the universality of them. According to the legend, King Wen of Zhou deduced the eight diagrams into sixty four diagram and wrote *The Book of Changes*. This book includes many dialectics thoughts, and

119

" – " (yang yao) and " – – " (yin yao) are used to illustrate two sides that are opposite and complementary to each other. In *Yi Zhuan* which was written in the Warring States Period, " – " is termed as yang, and " – – " as yin. By this, yin-yang theory and Eight Diagrams are integrated together, which enriches the dialectics thought, and the former becomes a more-perfected philosophical theory.

Five elements was originally called five materials or six places (there is a " grain" more in six places than in five materials, which indicated that the scholars then attached much importance to the notion of "food is the first necessity of people". While in the five elements, the "grain" is classified into "wood"). Later, the concept of five elements was abstracted. Furthermore, in order to emphasize their mutual relation and attribute of movement, the term "five elements" was determined instead of "five materials" or "six places".

Five elements generate and restrict each other, which is the relationship among them. The concept of five-element conquer appeared early in *Mo Zi* which says that none of the five elements can always conquer the rest. But which illustrated that the concept of five elements restrict each other existed in early time. While whether one restricts another in a certain order is controversial. Until the end of the Warring States Period, Zou Yan (340 B. C. – 260 B. C.) defined the order of five-element conquer. According to explanations in *Wen Xuan · Weidu Fu Zhu* quoted from *Seven Briefs* and recording of *Lv's Annals · Ying Tong*, *Zou Yan's Five-virtue Circle* was based on the sequence of five-element conquer which is derived from observation on

120

natural phenomena. Although the five-element generation and conquer do not reflect the essential contact of everything, it does explain the way everything relates. Especially the establishment of generation-restriction pattern reflects the basic law that everything relates, which is scientifically valuable.

Except the generation-restriction pattern, the significance of the five-element theory also manifested in the relation between five elements and number. For example, in *Zuo Zhuan* it says: "Things generate two, three, five··· so there are three celestial bodies in the sky, and five elements on the earth. In this cognitive process, "two" is a point, such as yin-yang which is a dichotomy taking "two" as a cardinal number. So is "five", such as five elements. In nature and society, the relation among things can be only summarized as advantages and disadvantages. The pattern based on number "five" is the most essential to explain the two kinds of relation. Any pattern based on numbers larger or smaller than "five" can not constitute the briefest pattern to express the two relations.

The essence theory, originally Taoism, was used to explain origin and unity of the world. Introduced in medicine, it became the foundation of TCM theory.

Lao Zi, the originator of Taoism, thinks that Tao, as the core of the world, has existed before the world formed. In Zhuang Zi, qi is considered as origin of everything, which actually defines Tao as essence. In *Gong Yang Zhuan*, it is put forward that archaeus should be the origin of heaven and earth. At the end of the Warring States Period, Song Xing and Yi Wen suggested essence being the vital part of qi, origin of everything. They clearly explained the Tao as qi. Qi is origin of the world, being everywhere. Everything tangible consists of qi. Essence is necessary for living things. Human bodies are combined with it. It changes and generates biological phenomena, spiritual consciousness and thinking activities. Then Xun Zi proposes that qi appears after the human body, which further confirms that spirit is the product of body and it cannot independently exist without body. Thus, essence theory actually was started by Lao Zi in the Spring and Autumn Period, and perfected till the Warring States Period when the materiality of qi or essence was affirmed and biological phenomena and spiritual consciousness were believed to be the product of body and the result of essence's movement.

At the end of the Warring States Period, on basis of the essence theory, Zou Yan combined the essence theory, the yin-yang theory and the five-element theory together, systematized them, and formed an independent theoretical system — the yin-yang and five-element theory. *Huang Di's Internal Classic* not only summarizes forefathers' medical experience and theories, but also adopts the yin-yang and five-element theory as its medical theoretical base and guiding ideology, establishing its own theoretical system and laying the foundation for TCM.

(2) *Huang Di's Internal Classic* is the mark of the establishment of TCM theoretical system

Huang Di's Internal Classic (*Internal Classic* for short) is the ear-

122

liest existing TCM theoretical monograph. According to *Han Shu · Yi Wen Zhi*, *Internal Classic* has been completed before the end of the Western Han Dynasty. It may be compiled in light of medical works since the Spring and Autumn Period and the Warring States Period. It mainly consists of extracts, so the content is multifarious and disorderly, some even inconsistent and paradoxical. The book now, though copy, revision and supplement, is totally different from the original version in content. The theoretical system may not have great changes.

The existing *Internal Classic* includes *Su Wen* and *Ling Shu* (aka Zhen Jing). Each has 9 volumes and 81 articles, altogether eighteen volumes and 162 articles. Through long-time circulation, the original book was incomplete. When Wang Bing of the Tang Dynasty recompiled the book, *Su Wen* lost 9 articles. Later 7 were found: *Tian Yuan Ji*, *Wu yun Xing*, *Liu Wei Zhi*, *Qi Jiao Bian*, *Wu Chang Zheng*, *Liu Yuan Zheng Ji*, *Zhi Zhen Yao*. Till Gao Baoheng of the Northern Song Dynasty revised it, *Ling Shu* was too incomplete to correct, so he only revised *Su Wen*. Gao also found *Ci Fa* and *Ben Bing* which were evidently different from the articles in *Su Wen*, so they were not included in it. Descendants compiled them as *Left Writings of Su Wen*. In the eighth year of Emperor Zhezong of Song Dynasty, in the book offered by Korea was the complete *Zhen Jing*. Since then a complete *Zhen Jing* appeared again, i. e. , *Ling Shu* of today.

Internal Classic is a medical theoretical monograph, covering a wide range of subjects, but still focuses on basic medical theories. Its contribution to medicine establishes medical theoretical system of

TCM. The main points of view are as follows:

① Succession of qi—monism thought. The basic viewpoint of Chinese ancient naive materialism which considers qi as the origin of everything and the differences are caused by diverse moving forms of qi. In *Internal Classic* it inherits the idea and says that the world comes up because of qi's motion. Qi fills the universe up and incessantly moves. It is due to the motion that there are change of seasons, renewal of everything and life and death. Humans are composed of qi and rely on it to keep normal geological activities. If the motion of qi is in disorder, biotic activities will be abnormal, which can cause diseases and death. So in *Su Wen · Ju Tong Lun*, it says diseases are caused by qi.

Since universe and humans are composed of qi, the motion of qi brings about changes of nature, as well as human biotic activities. Then qi can be considered as material basis of the unity of human beings and nature, which is the theoretical ground of correspondence between man and universe.

② Establishment of holism. The holism proposed in Internal Classic has two implications: one is the unity of man and universe; the other is the principle of integrity.

The former implication means that nature or universe and man exist together as a whole. Man is a component part of nature, which also has two meanings, i. e. , correspondence between man and universe, and similarity of them.

Correspondence between man and universe means that the struc-

124

tures of man and nature are similar. Man is a miniature of nature. Therefore, any structure of nature can be correspondently found in man; any change of nature can lead to correspondent reaction over man. So in *Ling Shu · Sui Lu Lun* it says that man and universe are complementary and correspondent. For example, a year can be divided into four seasons. As for plants, they sprout in spring, grow in summer, bear fruits in autumn and wither in winter. Man also reacts to different seasons. Besides, every time the solar terms alternate or the weather is cloudy or rainy, many chronic diseases will occur (especially lumbocrural pain).

Similarity of man and nature indicates that natural and demic changes have same or similar laws, according to which demic changes can be explained with the laws of changes in nature. For example, wind can bring about natural movement, like swinging trees and flying sand, and demic movements like convulsion and head shaking. Also, in winter coldness freezes water and contract objects. In human bodies, it can stagnate blood and cause cramp. Using natural phenomena to explain demic physiological and pathological phenomena solves the problem that they cannot be learned by intuitional approach. It is methodologically a great feature of TCM.

Both theories are based on the unity of man and nature as well as natural restrict over man. It is also a characteristic of TCM because it reflects the relation between man and nature to some extent.

The principle of integrity is that although man is composed of viscera, meridians, body, limbs, bones, five sense organs and nine orifices, they are a whole. If there is connection between human and the outside, the human body as a whole connects with the outside. In *Internal Classic* it says that man is a tiny world, an integrated system. The human body, with the five internal organs at the core, the heart as its dominator, meridians as roads all over, is an organic and holistic structure. When the outside acts on some part of the body, it is through meridians that the function spreads to the core part—headquarter made up by heart and five internal organs, and then to the whole body. When the body reacts to the outside, it is not partial, but under direction of the heart and five internal organs. Therefore, the reaction of any part is a partial manifestation of the systemic reaction. The disease of any position is a partial manifestation of the systemic disease. According to the principle, when a doctor copes with diseases, he or she must focus and treat them in light of the body's conditions. Of course, parts cannot be neglected. Only when the global-local relation is handled correctly, can the principle of integrity be applied wisely.

③ Establishing the guiding role of the yin-yang and five-element theory. *Internal Classic* takes the yin-yang and five-element theory which is based on the essence theory as guiding ideology and methodology throughout the whole medical theoretical system built by *Internal Classic*, learns the physiological and pathological process of human body in the view of yin-yang balance and interdependence and restriction as well as five-element inheritance and supervision guides clinical differentiation and treatment.

126

④ Creating a physiological structure centered by five internal organs and dominated by the heart — theory of visceral manifestation. In *Internal Classic* it emphasizes the integral principle of the human body and does not treat every component part averagely. It gives prominence to the five internal organs' functions and creates a five-internal-organ-centered, heart-dominated, and meridians-connected physiological structure, forming five physiological systems (cardiac system, pulmonary system, lienic system, hepatic system, nephric system) which are governed by mind to conduct vital activities. In *Ling Shu · Shi Chuan*, it says: "Five internal organs and six fu-organs are under domination of the heart." In *Su Wen · Ling Lan Mi Dian Lun*, it says: "all these twelve organs cannot be disharmonious. So if the heart is healthy, the other organs will be well; if not, then all the organs will be in danger." The quotes above stress the integrity of the human body and the dominant role of heart. It is on basis of the view that *Internal Classic* learns pathological phenomena and guides clinical differentiation and treatment.

⑤ Establishing etiological and pathological theories. *Internal Classic* denies the pathogenic effect of the supernatural, proposes that diseases are caused by the broken relation between the human body and its surroundings, or the broken coordinating relation inside the body, builds the etiological theory with nature, society, spirit and life as main factors, and emphasizes the significance of the endopathic cause (healthy atmosphere of the human body, i. e. ,disease-resistant function).

Internal Classic learns the pathological process on basis of etiological views, explains the occurrence of pathological phenomena with the break of the internal coordination relation of human bodies, and establishes pathological theory mainly about yin-yang disharmony, health-evil struggle, organ-qi disorder, qi-blood dysfunction, channel-qi blockage and so on.

⑥ Establishment of the basic principles of diagnostics and therapeutics. *Internal Classic* takes the yin-yang and five-element theory and the theory of visceral manifestation as basic views, and the four methods of diagnosis and differentiation as concrete content, and diseases are differentiated according to yin-yang, viscera, meridians, qi and blood and pathogenesis, identifies symptoms by yin-yang, four times, five internal organs, five colors, five tones, pulse manifestation and so on, and finally it constructs basic principles of diagnostics.

Under direction of the views and the methods above, *Internal Classic* proposes "prevention before disease onset", "preventing disease before exacerbating", "treating potential disease instead of existing disease"; early diagnosis and treatment, "treating unaffected part first"; "treating disease from root", handling symptom-root relation correctly; coordinating yin-yang, viscera-qi, and meridian-qi, regulating qi and blood, strengthening body resistance and eliminating pathogenic factors; ideas of therapeutics under guidance of adjusting measures to time, people and circumstances.

⑦ Establishment of basic principles of health preservation. Guided by correspondence among man and universe, six factors, moods and other pathogenic theories, *Internal Classic* puts forward basic principles of health preservation and disease prevention such as conforming to nature and weather, being modest and unselfishness, preventing diseases according to different times. It also proposes controlling diet and basic methods such as working and practicing to prevent disease and keep fit.

Internal Classic covers a wide range of content, from basic medical theory to the basic principles of clinical treatment, and establishes the framework of TCM theory. Until today, despite the great development, TCM theories are enriched and expanded in the light of the framework of TCM theoretical system designed by *Internal Classic*, without exceeding the scope of its theoretical system. Therefore, the completion of *Internal Classic* is the mark of basic establishment of TCM theoretical system.

Difficult Classic, also named *Huang Di's 81 Difficult Classic*, is another important medical theoretical work after *Internal Classic*. It consists of 81 medical problems. The time of completion is uncertain, maybe during the Qin-Han Dynasty or at the end of Eastern Han Dynasty. It is said that Bian Que wrote the book, but it is not credible.

In *Difficult Classic* issues are discussed such as sphygmology, meridians, viscera, process and prognosis of diseases, five acupoints, acupuncture manipulation, and so on. It not only inherits but develops the theories in *Internal Classic*. It puts forward "life gate", playing an important role in the development of San-Jiao theory and archaeus theory, having significant effect on the medical theories of later ages. Because of the great contribution to the establishment of TCM theoretical system, it has equal popularity with *Internal Classic*.

(3) *Shen Nong's Herbal Classic* establishes the theoretical system of traditional Chinese pharmacology (TCP)

Though *Internal Classic* proposes some principles on TCP and science of prescription, it is not a monograph on drugs and treatment. Moreover, *Internal Classic* is mainly about acupuncture treatment, so theories about pharmacology and science of prescription in this book are insufficient.

Shen Nong's Herbal Classic (Herbal Classic for short) is evidentially the first TCP monograph. It was completed around the first-year reign of King Ping of the Western Han Dynasty (1 A. D.). The writer is unclear. The original book had been lost, and the current version is divided in three columns collected from ancient herbal books by later generations.

Herbal Classic assembles TCP knowledge before the Qin-Han Period. It generalizes the functions of drugs with four properties and five flavors, explains pharmacological functions with cold, heat, tonification and purgation. According to toxicity and effects, drugs can be divided into three grades, higher, middle, and lower. Higher grade includes 120 drugs, which can tonify qi, and long-term use makes man light enough to be immortal; middle grade includes 120 drugs, which can tonify deficiency, and long-time use helps strengthen body and keep fit; lower grade includes 125 drugs, which is toxic and able to eliminate pathogens and cure diseases. The whole book records 365 kinds of drugs. *Herbal Classic* also puts forward the theory of compatibility and composition of monarch, minister, assistant and guide, with seven emotions. The pharmacology and science of prescription founded by *Herbal Classic* lay theoretical foundation for later development. Therefore, *Herbal Classic* marks the establishment of the basic theoretical systems of TCP and science of prescription.

Drug classification in *Herbal Classic* has little clinical and practical value, on which *Su Wen · Tiao Jing Lun* proposes different opinion. The function of higher-grade drugs reflects trend of pursuit for elixir and immortality during the Qin-Han Period. Most middle-grade drugs are mineral, not suitable to use. Drugs of lower grade, considered toxic and inappropriate for frequent use in *Herbal Classic*, can actually eliminate pathogens and cure diseases, and are commonly used in clinic.

(4) *Treatise on Febrile and Miscellaneous Diseases* establishes clinical medical theoretical system of TCM

Internal Classic is a monograph of medical theory. Although involving clinical medicine, it does not introduce diagnosis and therapy of certain diseases in detail. As to disease differentiation, *Internal Classic* proposes to differentiate diseases from pathogenesis, location and pathogen-resistance relation, but it is not specific, so the later generations cannot follow the example. *Shen Nong's Herbal Classic* is a monograph of pharmacology, recording basic principles of recipes and drug compatibility, while it does not elaborate usage, so problems still exist. Under this circumstance, *Treatise on Febrile and Miscellaneous Diseases*, as a

131

monograph of clinical medicine, fills the gaps mentioned above.

The book contains 16 volumes. According to history, it was written by Zhang Zhongjing, the Prefecture Chief of Changsha at the end of the Eastern Han Dynasty, and completed about the 15th year of King Xian of Han's reign (210 A. D.) Zhang wrote *Su Wen* (or *Ling Shu*) , *Jiu Juan*, 81 *Nan*, *Yin Yang Da Lun*, *Tai Lu Yao Lu*, *Ping Mai Bian Zheng*, and then compiled them together as *Treatise on Febrile and Miscellaneous Diseases*. He summarized achievements in clinical medicine before the Han Dynasty, and collected those of his times. But it was scattered and finally disappeared because of war soon after it was completed. Till the Jin Dynasty, by an Imperial physician Wang Shuhe's collection, it was integrated but soon lost again. Till the early stage of the Tang Dynasty when Sun Simiao compiled the *Invaluable Prescriptions for Ready Reference*, he was not able to see the book and said: "doctors of Jiangnan keep Zhongjing's prescriptions as secret and refuse to impart them. " Until Sun wrote *Supplement to Invaluable Prescriptions for Ready Reference*, he included *Treatise on Febrile and Miscellaneous Diseases* in it. When Gao Baoheng, Lin Yi and Sun Qi of the Northern Song Dynasty revised medical books, *Treatise on Febrile and Miscellaneous Diseases* has been separated into *Treatise on Febrile Diseases* and *Synopsis of Golden Chamber*.

Treatise on Febrile Diseases is a monograph of externally contracted heat diseases, including 10 volumes and 22 articles, setting 397 rules and 113 prescriptions. The book founded therapies and prescriptions of "six-channel differentiation" and theoretical system of clinical

132

medicine about differentiation and treatment, respected as the origina-tor of medical formulary. *Synopsis of Golden Chamber* had already been lost during Gao Baoheng revising medical books. Then according to *Synopsis of Golden Chamber and Jade Cover*, Sun Qi abandoned the first volume, divided the other two volumes into three, altogether 25 articles, 262 prescriptions, and renamed it as *Prescriptions of Golden Chamber*, i. e. , *Synopsis of Golden Chamber* of today. It is a mono-graph of miscellaneous diseases, creates theoretical system of clinical medicine about differentiation and treatment of the diseases based on the "viscera differentiation", and proposes three-factor etiological classification that despite thousands of diseases, their pathogeneses cannot exceed three kinds. In light of this, Chen Wuze of the Song Dynasty put forward "three-factor" doctrine.

The completion of *Treatise on Febrile and Miscellaneous Diseases* sets norms for the theoretical system of TCM clinical medicine, which enables the later generations to imitate. However, although people lat-er enrich and develop the clinical medical theories a lot, they still fail to exceed the differentiation-treatment system proposed by the book. Therefore, it marks the establishment of the theoretical system of TCM clinical medicine.

From *Internal Classic* to *Treatise on Febrile and Miscellaneous Dis-eases*, the TCM theoretical system is fully established. Though the later generations contributes a lot to TCM theories and achieves great suc-cess, as to theoretical system, they just enrich and perfect it without fundamental changes.

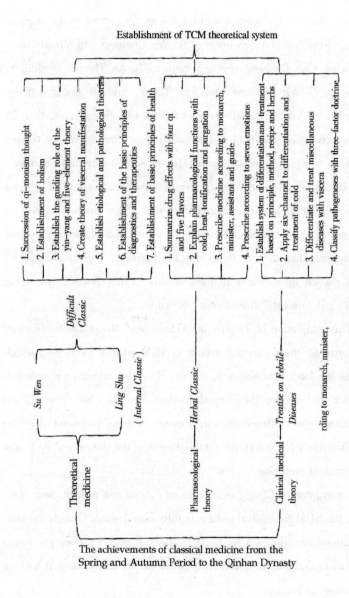

Figure 1. Establishment of TCM theoretical system

Yin, Yang and Five Elements

Yin-yang theory and five-element theory, yin-yang and five elements for short, is the naive materialism of Chinese classical philosophy and a kind of spontaneous dialectic ideology. Yin-yang theory and five-element theory is a universal law generalized from nature and society and one of the main philosophical ideologies used to learn natural and social phenomena.

The concepts of yin-yang and five elements had formed for a long time, but not until the end of Warring States Period when Zou Yan deduced the five elements and fused the essence theory, the yin-yang theory and the five-element theory together did the yin-yang and five-element theory form and become a popular philosophy. It is during this time that the development of Chinese ancient medicine came to a turning period when medical knowledge and experience had been rather rich and began to evolve into medical theories, while they needed the guidance of a philosophical ideology to process a great deal of medical materials and make them systematized and theorized. Under this condition, yin-yang and five-element theory which was most popular then was introduced as the guiding ideology and methodology of TCM theory, taking special position in TCM. Due to these reasons, people who learn TCM also have to learn and master yin-yang and five-element theory, or they cannot dig into and master theoretical system of TCM in depth.

After all, yin-yang and five-element theory, as an ancient philosophy with the deep brand of age, has some deficiency itself. Therefore, when we study it, it has to be analyzed from the perspective of dialectical and historical materialisms, absorbing essence and discarding dross, to serve medical practice better.

In TCM theories, yin-yang and five-element theory is mainly applied, while for the purpose of convenience, it is necessary to make separate introduction firstly and comprehensive discussion then.

Part I Yin-yang Theory

1. Basic concepts of yin-yang

(1) The formation of yin-yang's concepts

When the sun rises, one side of a mountain is toward the sun, bright and warm; the other side is back to it, dark and cold. The phenomenon is not specific to one mountain, but universally exists. Ancient people found the phenomenon and called the sunny side of the mountain as "yang of mountain" or "yang slope" and the shadier side as "yin of mountain" or "yin slope". It is the earliest use of yin-yang. In *Mountain and Sea Classic · Nanshan Classic*, it says that 185 km further to the east is a mountain named Niuyang Mountain which produces red gold (copper) at the yang slope and white gold (tin) at the yin slope. In *Master Lv's Spring and Autumn Annals*, it writes that the sun shines less space of bigger house and more space of higher platform. The yin-yang talked above is derived in light of sunlight. Toward the sun, the place receives sunlight is called yang; back to the sun, the place cannot receives sunlight is called yin. Thus, the original meaning of yin-yang is inferred only in light of sunlight. It is concrete and explicit instead of philosophically abstract meaning.

As long as there is a mountain, then the distinction between yin and yang of the mountain exists. If there is not, then the yin-yang of

137

the mountain does not exist. Therefore, ancient people regard them as two attributes that are opposite but exist in one mountain at the same time.

With the expansion of life and labor and accumulation of knowledge, people gradually realized the universality of two opposite attributes existing in one thing. For example, the universe consists of heaven and earth, heaven is light and thin, upward to be invisible; earth is heavy and thick, downward to be visible. A day is made up by daytime and night. The sun rises and shines brightly and warmly in the daytime; in the night, when the sun sets, the moon rises and brings darkness and cold. The seasonal change in a year brings about the alternation of cold and heat, because of which everything on the earth gains vigor and energy. The rain-shine change in weather prompts earth to thrive. Humans as well as animals are different in sex, which endows them with difference in characters and living habits, guarantees racial reproduction, and brings about prosperity in society and the animal world. Others like mountains being high or low, water being clean or dirty, things being light or heavy, locations being up or down, left or right, front or back and inside or outside, directions being east, west, south or north, movements being dynamic or static, rise or fall, fast or slow, advance or retreat, time being late or early, objects being big or small, wars being offensive or defensive, victory or defeat, biological phenomena being young or old, and life or death, all of these show that two opposite attributes or phenomena co-exist in one matter inseparably and make up a relatively independent

138

whole, which is a universal phenomenon. It is out of this that everything in the world emerges, develops and maintains the existence and development of the world. The ancient people used yin-yang to describe the two relevant and opposite attributes. Thus, the concrete concept of yin-yang, defined according to mountains' location to sunlight, is converted to an abstract one without concrete content, i. e. ,a philosophical category.

Yin-yang is the generalization about the relevant and opposite attributes of things or phenomena in nature and society. In *Ling Shu · Yin Yang Xi Ri Yue*, it says: "Yin-yang has names and is intangible. " It means that yin-yang has names and connotations instead of concrete image and signified. It is an abstract concept.

As an abstract concept, yin-yang has already existed before *Internal Classic* was completed, and it is used to explain some questions in medicine. For example, in *Zuo Zhuan*, Yi He analyzes causes of diseases with the six factors. He said: "The six factors are yin, yang, wind, rain, darkness and brightness. " Yin and yang here mean cold and heat. However, it is since *Internal Classic* that yin-yang is taken as an abstract philosophical concept, widely applied in medical theories and becomes an important component in TCM theoretical system.

Internal Classic, based on ancient people's understanding of yin-yang, introduce it in medial theories to learn and explain theoretical problems in medicine. In *Su Wen · Yin Yang Ying Xiang Da Lun*, it says that yin-yang is the Tao of heaven and earth, law of everything, parent of change, cause of life and death, origin of deities. Treating

139

diseases should seek the root. " Yin-yang is the most fundamental law of nature: everything can be classified by yin-yang and then outlined and summarized. The change of everything in the world is generated by yin-yang; the rise and fall of a life is caused by yin-yang; the root of the manifestation of biological phenomena exist in yin-yang, so diseases are caused by it and treating diseases should start from the root—yin-yang. *Internal Classic* inherits the viewpoint that yin-yang is the fundamental law of motion and variation, and draws the conclusion that it is also the fundamental law of medicine. In *Su Wen · Bao Ming Quan Xing Lun*, it says: "The various phenomena manifested by human life can not be separated from yin-yang. " In *Ling Shu · Bing Chuan*, it writes that as long as the law of yin-yang is understood, it is like a confusing problem about to be solved right away; it is also like a drunk person becoming sober immediately. *Internal Classic* takes yin-yang theory as methodology which enables people to think open-mindedly and wisely and solve problems effectively.

Internal Classic applies yin-yang theory to all aspects of medicine, including human anatomy, physiology, etiology, attack, pathogenesis and clinical diagnosis, differentiation, treatment and prevention, so yin-yang theory, as the ideology and methodology of TCM theoretical system, holds a special position.

(2) The integrity of yin-yang

Yin-yang is generalized from the two related and opposite attributes of matters and phenomena in nature and society, which proves that between yin and yang, there are contrariety and uniformity and

140

none is dispensable. Therefore, yin-yang can only exist in one relatively independent whole. Only when two matters or phenomena are related, and form an independent whole can the yin-yang relation be generated.

When conduct theoretical analysis, men and women are a pair of yin-yang relation. Since men and women are human beings and constitute the human society, this is the uniformity; while men and women have differences in sex, disposition, mentality, habits and social division of labor, this is the contrariety. It is because of these reasons that men and women compose a pair of yin-yang relation. But it does not mean that any man and any woman are related as yin-yang. If some man and a woman never have contact and relation with each other, then the yin-yang relation can not be established. In daily life, yin-yang relation is not limited between men and women, it also exists between men or between women, as long as there is some relation between them. For example, they complete a work together, have disagreement on something or participate same competition. As long as they are related, and form a relatively independent whole, the yin-yang relation is constructed. For another example, normally the hardness and the speed of an object are two concepts of different categories. They are unrelated and can not form yin-yang relation. However, they are both related with the object's temperature. If the object is moving with high speed, then it will inevitably lead to temperature variation which again can cause variation of hardness. Therefore, when studying an object's hardness variation during high-speed motion, since the temperature relates hardness and speed together, they compose a pair of yin-yang relation.

Therefore, whether there is a yin-yang relation between matters or phenomena depends on whether there is a unity of opposites between them, whether they are associated with each other, and whether they can form a relatively independent whole. Yin-yang relation only exists between concretely-related matters or phenomena and in one relatively independent whole. Without concrete relation and matters or phenomena existing in one relatively independent whole, there is not any yin-yang relation. This is the integrity of yin-yang.

(3) The relativity of yin-yang and the prescriptive nature of its attributes

① The relativity of yin-yang. On the one hand, it means that yin-yang itself is a relative concept, because it was originally defined according to mountains' position to the sun. One side of a mountain is toward the sun, and the other side must be back to the sun. If the sunny side does not exist, then the shadier side does not exist, either. The two sides coexist in one mountain, inseparable and comparative. Yin-yang can also be used to signify high and low temperature, cold and heat, fast and slow movement, dynamic and stationary, heavy and light objects, and quick and dull reaction, which are all relative concepts and coexist in comparison. For example, when we watch a game of the women's national volleyball team on TV, though the players are all taller than 1.8m, they do not give the audience this impression, because they are averagely tall. If a relatively short worker walks to them, then we become aware of that they are really tall. The comparison manifests their heights. It is said: "when you come to the Huangshan Mountain you do not climb it." It means that the view of the Huangshan Mountain is beautiful and incomparable; and the mountain is so high that it towers into the clouds. Climbing to the top of the Huangshan Mountain and standing in the cloud and mist is like exposure to a wonderland and is quite a view. Considering the altitude of the Huangshan Mountain, the Lotus Peak, also the highest one of the mountain, is only 1873 meters high. Compared with the Qinghai Plateau, Huangshan Mountain is over 1000 meters lower; compared with the Tibet Plateau, it is lower than the half, let alone to compare with the mountains on the plateaus. Even a swale is higher than the Huangshan Mountain. Actually, Huangshan Mountain broke out from low-altitude place, and nothing is comparable with it, so it seems especially high. The swales on plateaus, surrounded by mountains, seem very low, but actually higher than the Huangshan Mountain. Therefore, high and low, up and down, cold and heat, fast and slow, and fat and thin can be manifested only through comparison, without which these concepts are hard to establish. Once the conditions of comparison vary, so do people's impressions. Therefore, two attributes expressed by yin and yang only exist in comparison. They are relative, not absolute.

On the other hand, the second meaning of relativity is that yin-yang is an abstract concept instead of a concrete matter or phenomenon. When discuss concrete matters, the concrete contents that yin-yang denotes are ascertained according to problems under discussion. For example, if what we discuss is the position of an object, then the contents that yin-yang represents can be up and down, high and low, front and back, or inside and outside; if the discussion is about an object's motion in a certain circumstance, yin-yang may represent fast and slow, in and out, rise and fall, or dynamic and static; if we discuss the occurrence of diseases, yin-yang may represent evil and health, qi and blood, ying and wei, and so on. Therefore, the concrete contents that yin-yang denotes are ascertained according to problems under discussion. Yin-yang itself does not represent any fixed content or concrete matter or phenomenon.

In TCM books, yin-yang is often used to represent certain content, with different meanings under different circumstances. *In True Words of Golden Chamber*, it says: "Speaking of a person's yin-yang, the surface is yang and the inside is yin; as to a body's yin-yang, the back is yang and the belly is yin; as for yin-yang in viscera, the five internal organs are yin and the six fu-organs are yang." In other words, when the problems under discussion vary, the denotation of yin and yang also vary. In *Su Wen · Yin Yang Ying Xiang Da Lun*, it says that violent rage hurts yin and wild joy hurts yang. Here, yin refers to yin viscus, i. e. , liver, and yang refers to yang viscus, i. e, heart, which are different from previous yin-yang's meanings. In *Su Wen · Tiao Jing Lun*, it says that evil is generated by yin or yang. Those generated by yang are because of wind, rain, cold or summer heat; those generated by yin are due to diet and living habits, as well

144

as joy and anger. From the words it can be seen that the denotations of the three pairs of yin-yang are different. The former two pairs refer to pathogenic sites. "Generated by yin" means that diseases occur from the inner part—viscera; "generated by yang" means that diseases occur from the surface—skin. The later pair refers to pathogenic factors, i. e. , men and women's sexuality. The application of yin-yang in TCM books is widely, so that the meanings must be inferred from the whole.

The relativity of yin-yang also indicates judgments on the yin-yang attributes of a specific matter or phenomenon. For example, if the temperature range is 0℃ – 10℃ , then 0℃ is yin, and 10℃ is yang; if the range becomes 10℃ – 100℃ , then 10℃ is yin, and 100℃ is yang. 10 ℃ can either be yin or yang, which depends on the question under discussion. If the precondition varies, then the yin-yang attributes of matters or phenomena vary. In other words, the yin-yang attributes of concrete matters and phenomena are unfixed, relative, and they vary with comparison standards. Therefore, in *True Words of Golden Chamber*, the five internal organs are categorized as yin, and the six fu-organs as yang; while in the five internal organs, according to different locations, heart and lung are yang, and spleen, liver and kidney are yin; between heart and lung, heart is yang within yang, and lung is yin within yang; among spleen, liver and kidney, liver is yang within yin, kidney is yin within yin, and spleen is extreme yin within yin. There are all to explain the yin-yang attributes of the five internal organs in terms of comparative relation.

② The prescriptive nature of yin-yang attributes. Yin-yang is a relative concept. It does not refer to a certain matter or phenomenon, but determine the signified according to questions under discussion. However, the attributes of yin-yang are prescriptive. Once the scope of questions are settled, the two sides of this question and their yin-yang attributes are settled and unchangeable. For example, during the process of studying objects' temperature, those with higher temperature are yang, and those with lower temperature are yin; those with increasing temperature are yang, and those whose temperature drops are yin. When it comes to objects' motion state, those that move actively are yang, and those that move passively are yin; the dynamic ones are yang and the static ones are yin; those that move fast are yang and those that move slowly are yin; those that move upward are yang, and those that move downward are yin; accelerating ones are yang, and decelerating ones are yin. In the study of kinetic energy state, the hyperfunctional are yang and the hypofunctional yin; those in excitatory state are yang and those in inhibitory state are yin; those with gradual strengthened function are yang and those with gradual decreased function are yin. In the study of animals' sex, the male are yang and the female are yin; the fierce female animals are yang within yin, and the mild male animals are yin within yang. On these issues, the two sides of yin-yang are not interchangeable.

The yin-yang attributes are prescriptive. It is because the original connotation of yin-yang was concrete phenomenon, i. e. , mountains' position to the sun. Though yin-yang is abstracted later, its connotation

146

is not completely separate from the original one. Sunshine brings nature brightness, warmth, vigor and prosperity; without sunshine it means darkness, cold, death and silence of everything. Therefore, it is summarized that all those are bright, warm, upward, active, lively, brisk, outgoing, functional, sthenic, invisible, clear, growing, increasing, competitive, and so on, belong to yang; all those are dark, warm, downward, silent, passive, introverted, material, declining, visible, turbid, withered, decreasing, concessive, and so on, belong to yin. The features of yin-yang are all derived from its original connotations. When we analyze the attributes of certain matters or phenomena, we should, according to the attributes of yin-yang, make analogy with those of certain matters or phenomena, then draw conclusions, and classify them into yin or yang. For example, when we study the transparency of liquid, the clear, transparent and thin liquid is much closer to invisible and feels bright, so it belongs to yang; the turbid and thick liquid is closer to visible and feels dark, so it belongs to yin. As to the study of sex, no matter humans or animals, the female tend to be introverted, quiet, gentle and transigent, so they are yin; the male tend to be outgoing, active, fierce and aggressive, so they are yang. Due to the prescriptive nature of yin-yang attributes, when the issues discussed are determined, whether one side of the issue is yin or yang should be judged according to yin-yang's features and cannot be matched casually.

③ The relation of contradiction and yin-yang. Contradiction is also a unity of opposites and a relative concept instead of being specific to one certain matter or phenomenon. Its connotation must be determined according to questions under discussion. In these aspects, contradiction and yin-yang are same. However, the attributes of contradiction are not prescriptive and the two sides of it are interchangeable. Taking "up" and "down" as an example, either can be the spear or the shield, which does not affect the discussion. While in yin-yang, "up" can only be yang, "down" can only be yin, and they are not interchangeable. On this point, contradiction and yin-yang are different. The relativity of yin-yang is conditional and not radical, while that of contradiction is unconditional and radical. Therefore, the application of yin-yang is conditional while that of contradiction is not. Because of this, to take place yin-yang with contradiction is infeasible. Their concepts are different.

(4) The divisibility of yin-yang

Yin-yang is divisible, which means that yin-yang can be separated into yin and yang and the separation goes on without excluding yin-yang. In *Su Wen · Yin Yang Li He Lun*, it writes that if there are ten yin-yang, then it can be inferred to a hundred; if there are a thousand yin-yang, then it can be inferred to ten thousand. Ten thousand is a large amount and innumerable, but there is one key point. The sentence means that yin-yang can be separated infinitely, even till ten million, but there is only one essential method, i. e. , the method of yin-yang.

Yin-yang is separable to the minimum with yin-yang still included. For example, a magnet has N and S poles. According to "one divides into two", even if the magnet is divided to the minimum, as long as it is magnetic, it still includes N and S poles.

If an object is separable and each part has relative integrity, it indicates the levels of the object's structure. For example, in holography, any point of a picture, once magnified, is a complete picture again. For another example, the body structure is a combination of five physiological systems centered by the five internal organs. Every system is a relatively independent whole, composed by internal organs, fu-organs, body constituents, apertures and so on, which have their own relative independence. Each internal or fu organ has its qi and blood, body fluid, yin-yang and so on. The human body is constituted by different levels. Different physiological systems cooperate and coordinate with each other, form a rigorous and organic whole and maintain humans' biological functions.

2. The basic content of yin-yang theory

(1) The basic ideas of yin-yang theory

Yin-yang theory holds that the world consists of yin-yang which is in perpetual movements; the movements cause the appearance, development and variation of everything in the world; different forms of movements lead to diversity of everything; yin-yang is mutually dependent, opposed and restricted, which brings about growth-decline change and mutual transformation of yin and yang. On the method, yin-yang theory is "one divides into two". These are going to be discussed in relevant parts. Here only two questions are discussed as follows:

① Ideas of the balance theory. Yin-yang theory is a general law summarized from life, nature and social phenomena by ancients. In the ancient times, the social productive forces were so extremely underdeveloped that humans were not able to keep warm and full, rushing around for food and shelters. Under this situation, their biggest hope was to have adequate food and clothing, not daring to desire more. It was on this kind of economic basis that yin-yang theory came into being, which was also the social root where the balance theory grew.

Yin-yang theory was gradually perfected during the Spring and Autumn and the Warring States Period when many countries contended for hegemony. Under this circumstance, a weak country must seek balance of power to survive. Standing among other powerful countries, the weak countries had to be attached to them and created factors of containment among the seven powers so as to live in the narrow gap. Yin-yang theory was perfected during this time, so it was impossible not to be affected by the balance theory or the containment theory. Therefore, in yin-yang theory, when dealed with the relation between yin and yang, we used two methods — "balance" and "containment".

In nature, "balance" is also a basic way to keep things stable, such as the ecological balance. Fertilizer—plants—herbivores—carnivores constitutes a biologic chain, the balance of which is a necessary condition for their synchronous development. Animal carcasses and feces provide fertilizer for plants' growth, plants are fodder of herbivores, and herbivores become food of carnivores. Only when they are in balance can they develop synchronously. Any change of a link can cause synchronous reaction of other links. For example, drought leads to reduction of plants' output, which brings about hunger and death to herbivores. The number of carnivores is also going to reduce with it. It is through this way that nature regulates or controls the development of creatures, to restrict reproduction and increase and keep the ecological in balance.

In the human society, there must be a balance between sexes. If the balance is broken, it will become an unstable factor of society. Fortunately, under nature's control, the number of men and women just fluctuates in a small range and keep balanced on the whole. It is significant for social stability and humans' progress.

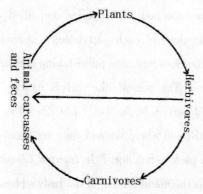

Figure 2. Ecological balance between plants and animals

Illustration: if plants reduce, herbivores will reduce because of shortage of fodder. Many carnivores will die of hunger, but their carcasses increase fertilizer and prepare conditions for increasing production in the next year. Plants increase,

151

so do herbivores and carnivores. But due to the limit of lands, the increase of plants is limited, so animals cannot increase infinitely, but only keep the balance between plants and animals

Internal Classic uses yin-yang theory to elaborate medical theory and agrees the viewpoints of the balance theory. In *Su Wen · Sheng Qi Tong Tian Lun*, it says that only when yin and yang are balanced can they be hidden inside and a person's spirit keep normal. It is also mentioned in *Su Wen · Tiao Jing Lun* that yin and yang meridians intersect at the shu-acupoint. Qi and blood get full in yang meridians and then go to yin meridians. After filled up in yin meridians, they will be transfused into yang meridians. Thus, qi and blood in yin and yang meridians are even and balanced, so as to keep human bodies in good condition. Once the body is supported and filled with average qi and blood, the functions of each part become normal, so the pulse condition of three portions and nine pulse-taking sites are same without excess or deficiency. The person like this is called "balanced person", i. e. ,normal person. In *Su Wen · Zhi Zhen Yao Da Lun* it says that, "Look over the site where yin and yang are excessive or deficient and regulate them back to balance. " In *Internal Classic*, it writes that yin-yang balance is the manifestation of the body's physiological condition, while the breakup of the balance is that of pathological condition. As a result, the key of treatment is to regulate yin and yang and restore the balance, and then the body's condition will be back to normal.

Internal Classic emphasizes yin-yang balance which is concerning

152

the scope of medical study. The aim of medicine is to protect human bodies and prolong life-span. The scope of medical study is limited between normal and sick people, making sick people recover. Yin-yang balance is necessary for health, so *Internal Classic* sticks to the ideas of the balance theory.

② Ideas dominated by yang-qi. The yin-yang theory is based on the balance theory, which does not mean that yin and yang are equally important. The attitude of *Internal Classic* is that yang qi is dominant. In *Su Wen · Sheng Qi Tong Tian Lun*, it says: "Yang qi is like planets and the sun. If the sun can not play its role, then the creatures in nature will die and the phenomena of rise and fall will disappear. Hence, the revolution of planets should be centered by the sun and let it shine and produce heat for the nature. *Internal Classic* stresses the importance of sunlight in nature, which is the primary reason that biological phenomena appear. Likely, yang qi is also dominant during the whole life of a person

Why yang qi is dominant in *Internal Classic*? It can be explained in several aspects as follows.

Firstly, it is due to ancient people's realization of the origin of lives. When the life originated, water was first created which prepared conditions for the origin of lives, but it was not enough to just have water, fire is necessary, too. Only with certain temperature, i. e. , when water and fire are compatible, can lives appear. Therefore, fire (yang qi) is a key factor.

Secondly, as for biological phenomena in nature, sunlight brings

153

creatures vitality, without which there would be no light and warmth. Then it is impossible for most plants to bud, grow, bloom and bear fruit, and the animals' lives would be threatened. Sunlight endows nature with a prosperous scene. In tropical and subtropical zones, plants and animals flourish; in the frigid zone, plants grow slowly or do not grow at all, and animals are sparse. These all show that sunshine and temperature, as well as yang qi are crucial to lives.

Thirdly, from the point of biological phenomena, the living and the dead people are same on morphological structure. While there is essential difference, the living people have biological phenomena but the dead not. Under the condition of the ancient times, the most easily found is that the dead are not breathing with lowering of temperature, which is a manifestation of no yang qi. The living people have yang qi, so they can breathe and have normal temperature, and drive all physiological functions; the dead ones do not have yang qi, so they stop breathing, lose temperature because of which all physiological functions stop. On this point, people's life and death depend on the existence of yang qi instead of the shape. It indicates that yang qi is significant for people and dominant in lives. Of course, only when yang qi is attached to the shape can the biological phenomena occur. Without the shape, yang qi has no meaning to lives.

Forthly, with regard to the death process, though death can be caused by various reasons, people will not die until yang qi is drained. The drain of yang qi is the direct cause of death. Only when some diseases like yin depletion, hemorrhage and sweating lead to the

154

drain of yang qi can death happen.

All above show that yang qi is importance to lives, so in *Internal Classic*, its content is dominated by yang qi, and this viewpoint is applied to explain physiological and pathological phenomena of human bodies. To emphasize yang qi's importance is not to deny yin qi's importance. In *Lei Jing Tu Yi*, it says: "Yin does not grow without yang, and yang do not form without yin. " "Single yin does not grow without yang, and single yang does not develop without yin", proposed by ancient men, also suggests the interdependence between yin and yang. They coexist as one and can not separate. In *Su Wen · Sheng Qi Tong Tian Lun*, it says: "The key of yin and yang is that when yang is compact, the body will be strong. If yin and yang are disharmonious, it is like spring without autumn, winter without summer. Their harmony can be called imperial grace. So if yang is intense and not compact, yin qi will be exhausted; if yin and yang are in balance, the mind will be kept in good condition; if yin-yang is separated, the vital essence will totally be lost. " This statement emphasizes the dominance of yang qi and the importance of yin-yang balance and interdependence. If yin-yang is separated, it will lead to death.

(2) Yin-yang taxonomy

Yin-yang theory is virtually a kind of taxonomy. In *Lei Jing · Yin Yang Lei*, it says: "Yin-yang, i. e. , one divides into two. " Zhang Jingyue thought that yin yang is dichotomy.

Internal Classic first proposed the proposition ——"Yin-yang is corresponding to signs". It means that things or phenomena in nature have specific appearances and signs, and they are corresponding to yin-yang. According to the relation, the things or phenomena in nature can be classified into yin and yang, which is called yin-yang taxonomy.

In light of yin and yang's attributes, yin-yang taxonomy makes an analogy with appearances of things or phenomena and classifies them into yin and yang. In *Su Wen · Yin Yang Ying Xiang Da Lun* it says: "Yang accumulates as heaven, and yin as earth; yin is static and yang restless; yin grows when yang arises, and yin hides when yang is restrained; yang turns into qi and yin forms shapes···Water is yin and fire is yang; yin flavor comes out from lower orifices, and yang qi from upper orifices; thick flavor is yin, and thin flavor yang within yin; thick qi is yang, and thin qi is yin within yang···" According to yin and yang's attributes, these are classified by analogies with some phenomena to illustrate the occurrence mechanism.

Relevant and contrary phenomena are ubiquitous, so yin-yang taxonomy has widely significance. Like add and subtract, multiply and divide in math, acting force and reactive force in mechanics, combination and decomposition in chemistry, and so on, all can be categorized into yin and yang.

Examples of yin-yang taxonomy

Attributes	Natural Phenomena	Spatial position	Motion state	Vital phenomena
Yang	heaven, sun, day, sunny	out, up, front, right	dynamic, rise, float, forward	grow, develop
Yin	earth, moon, night, rainy	in, down, back, left	static, fall, sink, backward	aging, mature

Attributes	Time	Form quality		Temperature		Luminance
Yang	early	intangible	function	warm	hot	bright
Yin	late	tangible	matter	cool	cold	dark
Attributes	Thickness	Transparency	speed	Function state		Weight
Yang	thin	pure	fast	excited	sthenic	light
Yin	thick	turbid	slow	restrained	declined	heavy

Attributes	Mechanics	Physical state		Electricity	Chemistry	Gravitation
Yang	acting force	gas	liquid	positive	decomposition	repulsive force
Yin	reactive force	liquid	solid	negative	combination	attractive force
Attributes	Density					
Yang	thin	sparse				
Yin	thick	dense				

Yin-yang taxonomy can also be applied to the human body. For example, the surface is yang and the inside is yin; the upper body is yang and the lower is yin; the back is yang and the belly is yin; the limbs are yang and the trunk is yin; the six fu-organs are yang and the five internal organs are yin; qi is yang and blood is yin; jin is yang and ye is yin; the upper orifices (eyes, ears, mouth and nose) are yang and the lower are yin. Other physiological and pathological phenomena of the human body can be classified into yin and yang.

The significance of yin-yang taxonomy lies in two aspects: one is to classify matters or phenomena in nature into yin and yang, which is helpful to explain them with yin-yang theory, including body structure and physiological or pathological phenomena. The other is to connect nature and the human body together through yin-yang taxonomy and to crystallize the theories, "unity of man and universe" and "correspondence between man and universe", which provides bases for the etiology and the pathogenesis of TCM.

The idea of yin-yang interaction between man and nature is one of the basic viewpoints of TCM theory, existing throughout every part of TCM theory, such as the theory of visceral outward manifestation, the meridian theory, etiology, pathogenesis, and theories of diagnosis, treatment and prevention in clinical medicine. All of them are based on the idea which is based on yin-yang taxonomy.

(3) The connection way of yin and yang

In *Internal Classic*, it puts up with the proposition——"separation and union of yin-yang", which is exactly the summarization of the connection way of yin and yang.

The proposition means that yin-yang can be separated and united. It is mutually repulsive and attractive, and the unity of opposites. It can be divided into two and united as one. Separation exists in union and the vice versa.

In *Ling Shu · Yin Yang Xi Ri Yue*, it says: "Yin-yang has names and is intangible, so it can be counted to ten and inferred to a hundred, a thousand, even ten thousand." It means that yin-yang is separable, i. e. , the separability of yin-yang. Except the taxonomy—"one divides into two", yin-yang can be divided according to "one divides into three", i. e. , "three yin and three yang". Three yang refer to taiyang, yangming and shaoyang; if united, they are called yi yang. Three yin refer to taiyin, juejin and shaoyin; if united, they are called yi yin. Yi yin-yang divides into threes yin and three yang which again can unite as yi yin-yang, i. e. , a whole. In fact, the separation and union of yin-yang is about the unity and opposition of yin-yang, i. e. , the relation of mutual restriction and promotion.

The yin-yang separation and union is dominated by union. Without union, there will be no unity of yin and yang, as well as the yin-yang relation. Only when there is unity between yin and yang and they coexist in one will the yin-yang relation form. In *Su Wen · Yin Yang Li He Lun* it says: "Yang gives yin-yang a name and yin is the governor of yin-yang", which emphasizes the coordination and unity between yin and yang, that is, yin and yang can only exist as one. However, the separation of yin-yang is also important. It means

159

mutual opposition and restriction of yin and yang. No separation, the union will be impossible. It is the separation and union of yin-yang that causes the movement of yin-yang and further the changes of things.

① Yin-yang interdependence and mutual rooting. The material world consists of yin and yang. Their movements present different patterns, so they lead to differences among substances and occurrence of everything. Hence, in matters or phenomena, there are inevitably yin and yang.

Either yin or yang exists on condition of the other's existence. Such as "up" and "down", "high" and "low", they are concepts drew from comparison. By comparison, we know something is "up", and "high" can be clearly showed. Without "down", there will be no "up"; without comparison between "high" and "low", "high" cannot be showed. Others like rise and fall, float and sink, dynamic and static, male and female, men and women, fat and thin, easy and hard, fast and slow, and so on, all concepts of relativity only exist in comparison. If one side does not exist, the other side itself cannot exist, either.

In *Su Wen · Yin Yang Ying Xiang Da Lun*, it says: "Yin is inside to restrain yang; yang is outside as manifestation of yin. " It emphasizes the interdependent relation of yin and yang. They can only coexist in a whole. In terms of the human body, yin is viscera and yang is the exterior manifestation of their functions. Viscera are attachment of vital functions that are showed outwardly; the vital functions showed outwardly are manifestation of viscera's functions. If viscera are good, the correspondent functions will be normal, and the vice versa. The exterior vital functions only manifest according to the viscera's condition. The viscera without functions cannot be called viscera, and functions without correspondent viscera, like a tree without root, do not exist. Therefore, either yin or yang exists on condition of the other's existence; if one side does not exist, the other side has no condition to exist. This is the yin-yang interdependence.

Yin and yang must depend on each other to grow and transform. Here it contains two meanings: one is that both yin and yang depend on each other to play its role; the other is that yin and yang can mutually transform.

For example, the machine tool needs power to function, or it is just a pile of useless iron. With power, it can make products and become useful. Since the machine tool and products are tangible, they are yin; the power is intangible, so it is yang. it indicates that yin's growth and transformation depend on yang. Electricity is a kind of common power. No matter hydroelectric or thermal power generation, the electric generator must be driven to generate electricity, so the generation of electricity must rely on the generator. It shows that yang's growth and transformation depend on yin.

Yin and yang can transform into each other. For example, while a ball is bouncing, with its rising, the kinetic energy gradually decreases and the potential energy increases; with its falling, the potential energy gradually decreases and the kinetic energy increases. Potential energy is yin, and kinetic energy is yang. the transformation of the two kinds of energy is an example of yin and yang's transformation.

Both yin and yang rely on each other to function and transform. It is the mutual generation, rooting and action between yin and yang. Yin can generate yang, and the vice versa. Under actual situation, they happen together. During growth and development of man, nutrients must be taken in from outside and transformed into components of the body to let it grow and viscera develop well, and at the same time, to promote the strengthening and perfection of vital functions. The process is rather complicated. Yin-yang interaction promotes strengthening and perfection of each other; their mutual transformation enable them to reach higher levels. In *Lei Jing Tu Yi* it writes: "Yin does not grow without yang and yang does not come into being without yin. " It emphasizes the mutual generation, rooting, and action between yin and yang. This is yin-yang interdependence.

The interdependence of yin and yang connects them as one, which is the unity of yin-yang. Without it, they cannot exist in a whole, so as not to construct the yin-yang relation, let alone the opposition and restriction of them.

② Yin-yang opposition and restriction. It is the second kind of relation between yin and yang, but it is the key factor to keep yin-yang in balance. Also, it is an essential element to preserve stable condition of things.

To let a matter persists, its inside must be stable. The level of inner stability decides the ability of persistence. For example, an ele-

162

ment's chemical activity depends on the atomic structure. An atom is composed of a nucleus with positive electric charge and one or more electrons with negative electric charge bound to the nucleus. The stability of the atomic structure rests with two conditions: one is that the value of the nucleus's positive electric charge of should be equal to the number of electrons with negative electric charge; the other is that the number of electrons on different electronic shells should satisfy certain amounts. If the two conditions above are met, the atom does not lose and get electrons easily. This kind of atomic structure has great stability. The atomic structures of inert elements satisfy the requirements above. Most elements' atomic structures only satisfy the first condition, i. e. , they reach charge balance instead of force balance. Therefore, they are in conditionally stable situation and have chemical activity, easily to lose or get electrons. Losing or getting electrons will break charge balance, transform the atom into an ion, and lose its stability.

The atom transformed into an ion by losing or getting electrons has active chemical properties, because the original charge balance has been broken. An ion cannot exist alone. It must bind with another ion with equal value of opposite charge, which satisfies charge balance and force balance and recovers its stable state. Different from the atomic structure, the electrons on the outermost shell are shared by two or more different atoms. Two or more different ions bind together and form the molecule of a compound, so as to return to the stable state.

In terms of the human body, to keep fit, it is necessary to stabilize the vital functions within normal range. In other words, yin and yang inside the body must be kept in normal balance. The destruction of the yin-yang balance means the disorder of yin-yang balance, i. e. , diseases. Therefore, in *Su Wen · Sheng Qi Tong Tian Lun* it says: "If yin-yang is in balance, the mind will be kept in good condition; if yin-yang is separated, the vital essence will totally lose. "

The facts above show that yin-yang balance is a common way and necessary condition for matters or phenomena in nature to keep stable state. Once it is broken, the stable state will disappear.

What kind of balance is the yin-yang balance? Generally speaking, it is a kind of relative, dynamic, constant and functional balance.

It is relative because between yin and yang imbalance within certain range is allowed. As long as the imbalance does not threaten a matter's stability, it belongs to yin-yang balance.

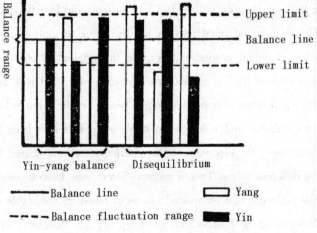

Figure 3. **Yin – yang relative balance**

Illustration: In the coordinate, within the balance range, the solid line is just theoretically equilibrium value. The dotted line is the permitted fluctuation range of balance. As long as yin and yang are within the range of dotted line, even if it is not balanced in value, it still belongs to balance since it does not endanger the stability of matters. Once yin or yang is higher or lower than the balance range, it is disequilibrium.

Speaking of matters' three states, generally water is solid under 0℃, liquid between 0℃ – 100℃, and gas beyond 100℃. Therefore, when the temperature varies between 0℃ – 100℃, the liquid state is quite stable. Only when the temperature is beyond 100℃ or under 0℃ will the liquid state be broken. Some matters are liquid only within small range and its liquidation temperature is almost close to the gasification temperature, so its liquid state is rather instable.

Human life can only keep normal under certain circumstances, beyond which it will be under threat. For example, the pH value of humans' extracellular liquid varies between 7. 35 ~ 7. 45, which has no influence on vital functions. Once the fluctuation range beyond the normal, it will cause acidosis or alkalosis. Thus, it will be impossible to maintain the normal vital activities.

The examples above indicate that yin-yang balance has an allowable range to fluctuate. Within it, even if yin and yang are not balanced, it will not endanger matters' stability. As a result, it is still considered balanced, which is the meaning of relative balance.

The significance of relative balance lies in the expansion of stability. If yin-yang balance allows larger range of fluctuation, it will not

165

be broken easily. If the range is smaller, the stability will be weaker and be destroyed easily. The human body is adaptive to surroundings, which is taken as the reflection of the permitted range of yin-yang balance. When there are changes, it will not harm to the body if the changes are not beyond the adaptive capacity. Under the contrary condition, the changes will give rise to such harms as frostbite, burn, dehydration, drowning and infectious diseases. The adaptability—— the stability of yin-yang balance——is the ability to resist exogenous evils.

The balance between yin and yang is dynamic, which has two aspects of meanings: one is that it is achieved during the continual movements of matters or phenomena; the other is that the balance range or point of yin-yang balance varies at different moving stages of the matters or phenomena.

The world is in continual movement, so are the matters and phenomena. Under the circumstances, yin-yang balance can only be obtained during the course of movements and changes. The periodical variation of a year causes the periodical change temperature, while the body temperature of man can only be controlled around 37℃. Therefore, the functions of heat production and dissipation have to make changes corresponding to different seasons. Heat production is intensified in winter and dissipation is strengthened in summer so as to keep the body temperature within a normal range. For another example, when an athlete is doing floor exercises, he/she has to run, jump, roll, somersault, and so on, as well as to make various postures. Once

166

he/she is careless with the balance, it causes faults. Different from the static condition, to keep balance in motion, the athlete has to adjust the center of gravity and correct postures. In the entire exercises, the center of gravity moves in accordance with actions to ensure accuracy and elegance. All indicate that moving matters or phenomena make self-adjustments in motion to achieve balance.

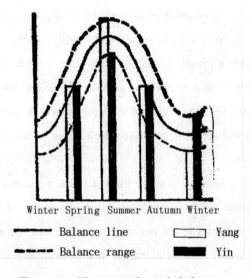

| | Balance line | | Yang |
| | Balance range | | Yin |

Winter Spring Summer Autumn Winter

Figure 4. Yin – yang dynamic balance

Illustration: The figure takes four seasons as an example to illustrate yin-yang dynamic balance. In the seasonal changes, yin and yang will change correspondingly. Yang is the most excessive at the summer solstice and yin is the most excessive at the winter solstice. Therefore, the fluctuation of yin and yang presents hyperbolic curves. Moreover, yin and yang have its own fluctuating curve (not shown in the figure). The fluctuation range of yang qi is larger than that of yin qi.

For moving matters or phenomena, their positions of yin-yang balance are not fixed, but change with movements. A person, from birth to death, goes through growth, maturity and senility. The nature of the different stages is the balance between growth and senility. Before middle age, growth is dominant, presenting itself as growth and development, and the point of balance is close to the growth; during the middle age, growth and senility come into balance with unapparent trends, manifested as maturity in all aspects, and the point of balance is in the middle of growth and senility; in the stage of senility, the trend of growth declines, while senility is increasingly dominant, and the point is close to senility. Therefore, with regard to a man's whole life, the position of yin-yang balance is not fixed, but varies at different stages of the life, which is the second meaning of dynamic balance.

Yin-yang balance is also a kind of constant balance, which is to say that during certain periods or stages, the range of yin-yang balance is a constant. Even if yin and yang are balanced, greater or less than the constant value is abnormal. It is normal only within the constant range. For example, the amounts of various compositions in the human body are constants. The proportion of plasma is $1.024 \sim 1.029$, the number of erythrocytes in a male's blood is $4 \sim 5$ million $\cdot$ mm^{-3} and in a female's blood is $3.5 \sim 4.5$ million $\cdot$ mm^{-3}. To maintain the normal physiological function, various compositions in the human body must reach the average level, or it will be affected.

Illustration: Only if yin-yang balance reaches to the permitted range of normal value can it will be normal balance. Beyond the range, though yin and yang

168

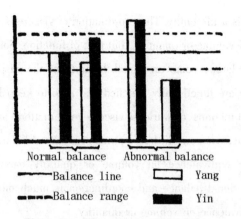

Normal balance   Abnormal balance

━━━━ Balance line   ▭ Yang

■ ■ ■ Balance range   ■ Yin

Figure 5. Yin – yang constant balance

are balanced, it is abnormal.

It is same for the yin-yang balance in the human body, which has to be within the normal range. In different ages, the constant values are different, but to the people at similar or same age, the values are approximate. Except for age, the constant of yin-yang balance is also involved with sex. At present, it is impossible to do the quantitative analysis of yin-yang and to learn the accurate values of yin-yang balance in the age or sex group, but there is a rough concept of quantity. For example, among patients of yin-yang deficiency and qi-blood deficiency, there are low-level yin-yang balances. Though their yin and yang are balanced, they are abnormal. Therefore, in clinical treatment, only to regulate yin-yang for the purpose of balance is not enough. Actually, it is necessary to make yin-yang balance reach the average level, which can help eliminate the pathosis.

Yin-yang balance is also functional, not necessarily quantita-

169

tive. Human is a life entity. The coordination of viscera is not due to e-quivalence of volume or quantity, but that of function. Some viscera in the body are large, some are small. In spite of the disproportion on volume, they are functionally matched and able to keep life functions normal. The functions of various viscera and matters are different, some are great, some are little. To pursue functional balance and coordination, the equivalence on volume or quantity cannot be satisfied. The functional balance and coordination is much more important than the equivalence on volume or quantity.

In nature or the human body, to maintain yin-yang balance, there exists a kind of automatic regulation mechanism which is the yin-yang opposition and restriction.

Yin and yang are opposite concepts with one side restricting the other. The degree of restrictive power that one side exerts on the other is inversely proportional to its own rise and fall, and directly proportional to another's. In other words, when yin and yang lose balance, the restrictive power from the weaker side is greater than that from the opposite side; as the gap of power becomes wider, the restrictive power from the weaker side will be greater and that from the opposite side will be weakened and disappear at last. It is through the mutual restriction that the yin-yang balance is maintained. In *Lei Jing Tu Yi*, it writes: "Motion to extreme should be slowed by motionlessness, and excessive yin should be conquered by yang. " "Motion to extreme" and "excessive yin" are description of yin-yang's rise and fall. "Slow" and "conquer" are description of the degree of restrictive power,

170

i. e. , the weaker side can exert greater restrictive power on the oppo-site side. It indicates that the degree of restrictive power that one side exerts on the other is inversely proportional to its own rise and fall. It is the manifestation of the law that things turns into their opposites when they reach an extreme, and also the major method to keep the balance.

The mutual generation of yin and yang also plays a part in main-taining the balance. It is in direct proportion to its rise and fall.

Yin-yang balance is relative, which means that yin and yang fluctuate around the balance point within a permitted range. The fluc-tuation is caused by the mutual generation and restriction of yin and yang which manipulates the range.

The regulation of body temperature includes two processes: heat production and dissipation, which ensures that the temperature is maintained around 37℃. In fact, body temperature is the balance point of heat production (yang) and heat dissipation (yin). Human physiological activities, as well as exercises will produce heat to ele-vate temperature. At the same time, sweating, radiation of heat and air convection can dissipate the inside heat to lower temperature. It is the interaction of heat production and dissipation that the body temper-ature can be kept around 37℃. They can be regarded as a pair of yin and yang. The body temperature is the place where yin and yang reach the balance. The permitted fluctuation range of normal body tempera-ture is that of yin-yang balance. In order to keep yin-yang balance within the permitted range, the interaction, i. e. , mutual generation or restriction, of heat production and dissipation must be harmonious and unified, and thus the body temperature can be normal. In the cases of diseases, due to dysfunction of temperature regulation, the balance point of heat production and dissipation skews and go beyond the normal range, so the elevation or reduction of body temperature manifests. If the mechanism of yin-yang regulation is in normal condition, or recovers after treatment, the human body can regain balance and health via yin-yang restriction.

(4) Yin-yang's modes of motion

Yin and yang are the unity of opposites. They not only mutually depend on, generate, root and act on each other, but also oppose, restrict and fight each other, which causes yin-yang's motion. The modes of motion, in terms of yin-yang's mutual conditions, are manifested as growth and decline as well as transformation of yin and yang; in terms of relation of matters and their surroundings, these modes are manifested as rise and fall as well as exiting and entering of yin and yang.

① The growth and decline of yin and yang. Yin-yang balance is relative and dynamic, which is reached through the course of movement. Therefore, in actual situation, yin-yang balance always fluctuates around a central point within a certain range. It is called growth and decline of yin and yang, i. e. , growth of yin and decline of yang, or growth of yang and decline of yin.

The fluctuation is like tide, moving forward with rise and fall. Yin and yang always move in opposite directions, i. e. , yin rises and yang falls, yang rises and yin falls. They keep balance during move-

172

ments. Yin and yang alternatively grow or decline and they will go on and on, which can be described by a unit called growth-decline wave.

Taking the nature as an example, sprouting in spring and growing in summer are growth of yang and decline of yin, and harvesting in autumn and storing in winter are the other way around. They make up one year. For plants, this is a growth cycle. From the first yang that begins at 11:00 pm to the full yang at noon is growth of yang and decline of yin; from the first yin that begins at 1:00 pm to the full yin at midnight is just the opposite. They make up a day and become a basic unit of one month or one year. A man, from birth to prime, mainly grows strong instead of getting old, so this is the growth of yang and decline of yin in the body; and it is the opposite condition from prime to old age. They altogether constitute a man's life. Consequently, a growth-decline wave consists of two parts: growth of yin and decline of yang, and growth of yang and decline of yin.

There are two forms of yin-yang's growth and decline—the normal and the abnormal.

The normal yin-yang's growth and decline accord with the general rules of development in nature. They have two features: one is that the growth and decline only occur within a permitted range of the yin-yang balance; the other one is that the process includes two parts—growth of yang and decline of yin, and growth of yin and decline of yang. Yin and yang are not balanced at particular point, but as a whole they are.

Taking the example of the length of day and night to explore the relation of yin-yang growth and decline, day is yang and night is yin. After the winter solstice, day becomes longer until the summer solstice when day is 6 hours and 12 minutes longer than night (calculated in Hohhot). After the summer solstice, day becomes shorter till the winter solstice when night is longest, about 5 hours and 22 minutes longer than day (calculated in Hohhot). From the winter to summer solstice, day becomes longer and night shorter, so it is decline of yin and growth of yang; from the summer to winter solstice, day becomes shorter and night longer, so it is decline of yang and growth of yin. In a year, only on spring equinox and autumn equinox will the day and night be equal. In the half year, from the spring equinox to autumn equinox, day is longer than night, i. e. , excess of yang; in the next half year, night is always longer than day, i. e. ,excess of yin. on the summer solstice, day is the longest and night the shortest, i. e. ,yang extremity; on the winter solstice, night is the longest and day the shortest, i. e. ,yin extremity. The fluctuation range of day and night is almost 12 hours, but it is normal. Therefore, this is the permitted fluctuation range of yin-yang balance (day-night balance). Though the day-night length of 365 days in a year is different, on the whole, either day or night occupies half of the time. Therefore, yin and yang are balanced overall.

Illustration: In the coordinate axis, the ordinate represents time (in hours), the left-side values represent time D-value of day and night, the right-side values represents length of day and night. The abscissa represents seasonal changes. In the figure, the solid line is day curve, i. e. ,growth and decline of yang qi; the

174

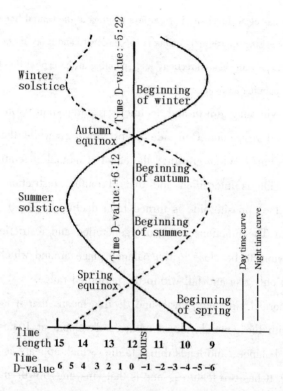

Figure 6. **Day and night time difference curve in Hohhot area**

dotted line is night curve, i. e. ,growth and decline of yin qi. At the summer solstice, day is 6 hours and 12 minutes longer than night; at the winter solstice, night is 5 hours and 22 minutes longer than day. In a year, summer solstice is yang extremity, and winter solstice is yin extremity, which are two yin-yang transition points of a year. Through summer or winter solstice, the rise and fall of yin and yang inverse. Other times are all yin-yang growth and decline with only change in the speed of rise and fall instead of inversion of rise and fall. In the figure, it is clear that yin-yang transformation is intermittent, and it occurs in the form of sal-

175

taiton and has clear direction, i. e. , always pointing at the central line of yin-yang balance; yin-yang growth and decline is successional, and it occurs in the form of gradual change with vague direction, i. e. , pointing at the central line before passes it and pointing away after passes it.

The yin-yang growth and decline is resulted from its mutual generation and restriction. One side keeps growing, while the opposite keeps declining. While growing, the effect of mutual generation on the opposite side is intensified and that of mutual restriction is weakened. So the opposite side is turned from decline to growth, and the vice versa. The functions of mutual generation and restriction control yin and yang to be close to the balance place around which yin and yang can only rise and fall within the permitted range.

Abnormal yin-yang growth and decline means that it is not consistent with the general rule of nature's development. It destroys the yin-yang balance, and leads things to die, which appears as pathological state. It has two features: one is that yin-yang growth and decline exceeds the permitted fluctuation range of yin-yang balance and moves away, which finally results in destruction of yin-yang balance and unstable state of matters and phenomena; the other one is that it cannot make up a complete growth-decline wave, with only decline of yin and growth of yang or decline of yang and growth of yin, which finally results in excessive yang and deficient yin or excessive yin and deficient yang, i. e. , yin-yang dissociation. Looking the whole process, yin and yang are impossible to reach balance because they cannot construct a complete growth-decline wave.

176

In terms of human bodies, abnormal yin-yang growth and decline only appears in diseases. A patient of wind-heat, stroke by yang evil, has excessive yangqi. At the start, it is just yang excess and yin has not been impaired. Then yinqi gets impaired and leads to yang excess and yin deficiency. Without appropriate treatment, the patient's condition will deteriorate, and yangqi will be more excessive and yinqi more deficient. At last, yang grows to extreme and yin exhaust. Exhausting inside, yin does not defend for yang, and yang does not function for yin, then yang qi exhausts outside, which leads to yin-yang dissociation and death.

The reason of abnormal yin-yang growth and decline is that the mutual generation and restriction of yin-yang become abnormal. The force of yin-yang mutual restriction is in direct proportion to the prosperity and decline of yin and yang, while the force of yin-yang mutual generation is in inverse proportion to it, which gives rise to the strong oppressing the weak. The strong get stronger and the weak get weaker. Yin and yang move away from the balance place and finally dissociate, so abnormal yin-yang growth and decline cannot forms a complete wave.

The abnormal yin-yang growth and decline can also be caused by external factors. Though the function of yin-yang mutual generation and restriction is normal, the external force is still more powerful than the regulating ability of yin-yang itself, so the yin-yang growth and decline moves away from the balance place. Under this condition, as long as the external force is weakened or the external evil is dispelled, yin and yang can reconstruct the balance though autogenous regulation.

②Yin-yang transformation. When move to certain extent, yin and yang respectively transform into its opposite side, i. e. , yin transforms into yang or yang transforms into yin, which is called yin-yang transformation.

Different from yin-yang growth and decline, yin-yang transformation has four features: firstly, yin-yang transformation causes changes of yin-yang's attributes, i. e. , qualitative change; secondly, the transformation of yin and yang is conditional, and it cannot happen at anytime; thirdly, its occurrence is discontinuous and in the form of saltation; forthly, it is directional, and they transform towards the place of yin-yang balance.

Yin-yang transformation causes changes of yin-yang attributes, i. e. , yin transforms into yang and yang transforms into yin. Yin-yang growth and decline only causes quantitative changes. Yin is still yin and yang is still yang, no changes in yin-yang attributes. From the graph of one-year yin-yang growth and decline, it can be seen: from the winter solstice, yang qi grows, and day becomes longer until the summer solstice; from the summer solstice, yinqi grows and night becomes shorter until the winter solstice. From the winter to the summer solstices is decline of yin and growth of yang. on the graph, it changes slowly from the start and then rises perpendicularly and then gets slow again; from the summer to the winter solstices is decline of yang and growth of yin. On the graph, the curve is smooth at the beginning and then falls straightly and gets smooth again. These indicate that in the

178

course of yin-yang growth and decline, there is only quantitative changes instead of qualitative changes. Winter and summer solstice are two yin-yang transition points. It is decline of yin and growth of yang before summer solstice, and decline of yang and growth of yin after summer solstice, and vice versa before and after the winter solstice. By the summer and the winter solstices, yin-yang growth and decline convert. By the summer solstice, yangqi firstly rises and then falls; by the winter solstice, it firstly falls and then rises. Rise is yang, and fall is yin. Therefore, after the summer solstice, yang converts to yin, and after winter solstice, yin converts to yang. It shows that the attributes of things changes. Consequently, yin-yang transformation causes the changes of yin-yang's attributes, i. e. ,qualitative changes.

Yin-yang transformation takes place conditionally, in *Internal Classic*, the conditions of yin-yang transformation are usually described by seriousness, extreme, and excess. These three words have similar meanings which suggest that only when movements or changes develop to extremity can yin and yang transform. In a year, yin and yang only transform at the summer and the winter solstices. The summer solstice is extremity of yang excess and the winter solstice is extremity of yin excess. When yang reaches extreme, it necessarily transforms into its opposite——yin; when yin reaches extreme, it will also transform into yang. In terms of the human body, when growth and development reach extreme, it begins to grow old, which is also a yin-yang transformation. While yin-yang growth and decline happen all the time, so it is unconditional.

In a year, yin-yang transformation only happens on the winter and the summer solstices. It's discontinuous and sudden and ends instantly. Therefore, yin-yang transformation occurs always in the form of saltation. The beginning means the end, because it is completed instantly. While yin-yang growth and decline is continuous and gradually proceeds for a long time until the appearance of yin-yang transformation, and then the yin-yang growth and decline of opposite direction begins. As a result, it is continuous and gradual, showed in the way of gradual change. The end cannot be seen except the change of growth-decline forms.

Yin-yang transformation is directional, i. e. , under normal circumstances, it is always towards the yin-yang balance place. When yin-yang growth and decline reaches the extreme which is the limit of the permitted fluctuation range, a further growth or decline will inevitably ruin the yin-yang balance. It is at this moment that yin-yang transformation occurs. It reverses the direction of the growth and decline and points at the yin-yang balance place. When yin-yang growth and decline has not passed the balance place, it points at that, but once it passes the place, the direction it points at is opposite the place. It can be concluded that yin-yang growth and decline is similar to inertial motion. Its direction does not always point at the balance place, but regulates by yin-yang transformation so as not to destroy the balance. Therefore, in light of the forms of yin-yang movements, the aims of transformation are clear. Tending to yin-yang balance is the main motion forms for yin-yang to keep balance.

180

Yin-yang transformation shows by the way of saltation, while the process of saltation has two forms. Generally speaking, it is always in succession with yin-yang growth and decline and takes place on the basis of it. For example, the yin-yang transformation of the winter and the summer solstices are the outcome when yin-yang growth and decline develops to certain extent. People who die of old age and diseases have changes of yin-yang growth and decline before the death. Only when the changes develop to some extent can they cause death. The saltations are all consequences of the gradual change of yin-yang growth and decline, which is consistent with the general rule in nature. However, sometimes yin-yang transformation is not in succession with yin-yang growth and decline. It occurs independently instead of on the basis of yin-yang growth and decline. For instance, people or creatures suddenly die from earthquake, flood, or other accidents. In terms of one individual, the yin-yang growth and decline has not reached the degree that can cause yin-yang transformation (death). It has nothing to do with yin-yang growth and decline, but an accidental coincidence.

Yin-yang transformation is resulted from yin-yang generation and restriction. Yin-yang restriction is in direct proportion to growth and decline of the restricting side, and in inverse proportion to that of the restricted; yin-yang generation is in direct proportion to the growth and decline of the promoting side, and in inverse proportion to that of the promoted. According to these principles, during the yin-yang growth and decline, when one side falls to the minimum of the permitted fluctuation range, it inevitably will exert strong restraint power on the opposite side, while the promoting power will recede to the minimum and force the opposite side to reverse from increase to decrease; when the other rises to the maximum, the restraint power has reduced to the weakest degree while the promoting power enhances to the maximum and urges the opposite side to reverse from decrease to increase. In the course of yin-yang growth and decline, the rising side becomes the falling one, while the falling side turns to the rising one, which enables the yin-yang growth and decline that has got away from yin-yang balance to reverse and move to the balance place. This is yin-yang transformation.

When the yin-yang restriction is malfunctioning and losing control of yin-yang growth and decline, it cannot cause the reversion, and it will bring about abnormal yin-yang growth and decline as well as transformation. On the human body, it is only showed in pathological state.

③The dialectical relation of yin-yang growth and decline and yin-yang transformation. Yin-yang growth and decline and yin-yang transformation are two motions of yin-yang. They are caused by yin-yang generation and restriction, and making up a complete state of motion altogether. To keep yin-yang in constant movements maintains yin-yang balance as well as stable state of matters or phenomena. Yin-yang growth and decline and yin-yang transformation together exist as a whole, use and restrict each other. They are a pair of yin and yang.

Generally speaking, yin-yang transformation is based on yin-yang

182

growth and decline. Only when yin and yang grow or decline to some extent can yin and yang transform. If they grow or decline beyond the limit and do not transform, it will definitely destroy the yin-yang balance. The limit of yin-yang growth and decline is the condition of yin-yang transformation, as well as the maximum fluctuation range of yin-yang balance. The fluctuation within the range will not endanger yin-yang balance; while once it goes beyond the range, it will.

Yin-yang growth and decline happens on the lower basis of yin-yang transformation. Anything's structure is hierarchical. Higher levels consist of lower ones which are made up of levels below. Every level is complete in structure, comprehensive in function, and independently exists as a unit under certain condition. The yin-yang growth and decline on the higher level is in fact the result of the yin-yang transformation on the next level. Since the component units of the next level orderly transform from yin to yang, then on the higher level yin declines and yang grows; yang transforms into yin, and then on the higher level yang declines and yin grows. This is the mutual-use relation of yin-yang growth and decline and yin-yang transformation. Yin-yang transformation limits the range of yin-yang growth and decline not to develop infinitely, so as to keep yin-yang balance; yin-yang growth and decline separates yin-yang transformation not to occur successively, so as to make the development of matters present different stages and is relatively stable. This is the mutual restricting relation of yin-yang growth and decline and yin-yang transformation.

Mutual use and mutual restriction of yin-yang growth and decline and yin-yang transformation are their dialectical relation of the unity of opposites.

(5) Yin-yang ascending, descending, exiting and entering

A thing contains yin and yang which denote the integrity of matters, i. e. , relatively independent units.

In a relatively independent whole, yin-yang moves ceaselessly, which causes yin-yang growth, decline and transformation. Yang governs ascending, and yin governs descending; yang is up and yin is down. Yang above necessarily joins yin below, because yinqi inhales downwards; yin below must joins yang above , because yangqi evaporates upwards. yangqi descends and yinqi ascends, which cause yin-yang growth and decline and accomplish things' birth, growth, maturity, oldness and death, as well as sprout, growth, bloom, harvest and store.

Anything is relatively complete and independent, but it always lives in concrete environments and acts as the component. Therefore, it acts on the surroundings, so does the surroundings act on it. In the yin-yang system, yin-yang is not exclusive, but relates the outside extensively. For example, a man has to take food and air from the outside, and also expel wastes. At the same time, external changes act on the human body; similarly any change of the human body will do the same to the surroundings. Since yin-yang is an open system, it will definitely exchange matters and information with the outside, which is the exiting and entering movements of yin-yang. Therefore, in *Su Wen · Liu Wei Zhi Da Lun*, it says: "Without exiting and entering, there will be no birth, growth, maturity, oldness and death; without ascending and descending, there will be no sprout, growth, bloom, harvest and store. Therefore, no viscera don't have ascending, descending, exiting and entering. "

(6) To discuss Yin-yang theory according to Tai ji diagram

Tai ji diagram is the ancients' summary of the yin-yang theory. It includes the main content of the theory. Here is the general explanation of the yin-yang theory according to Tai ji diagram.

Tai ji diagram is around, and equally divided into two tadpole-shaped parts by the curve " ~ ", which is called yin-yang fish. In the yin-yang fish, the big end is head and the sharp end is tail. Two parts are separately painted with black and white isto express yin and yang. On the head of the black yin-yang fish is a white dot, and on the head of the white yin-yang fish is a black dot. They are called small heart or eye. Thus a Tai ji diagram is constituted.

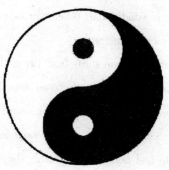

Figure 7. Tai ji digaram

①Tai ji diagram is a circle, divided into black and white. Black is yin and white is yang. They exist in a circle, which indicates that yin and yang exist as a whole.

②In the diagram, the areas of yin and yang are equal, which indicates that yin and yang are balanced.

③The circle is equally divided by the curve " ~ " instead of a straight line, which shows that yin and yang are moving ceaselessly.

④In the diagram, there is a black dot on the head of the white yin-yang fish, and a white dot on the head of the black one, which illustrates that yin has yang and yang has yin, yin and yang are separable and mutual-rooting.

⑤The straight line that goes through two dots and the center is the diameter of the big circle as well as that of each small circles of yin and yang. It is the extremity of yin and yang. The transformation of yin and yang starts from the two ends of the line, i. e. , extreme yin generates yang and extreme yang generates yin. It means that the yin-yang transformation is conditional. When yin or yang develops to the extremity, then they can transform.

⑥Yin-yang transformation starts from two ends of the straight line that goes through the circle center and two dots. Yin and yang separately transform into its opposite, i. e. , yin transforms into yang and yang transforms into yin. Therefore, in yin-yang movements, yin-yang fishes's heads recede and tails move forward. They move in a circle around the center of Tai ji diagram which is manifested as yin-yang rise and fall.

⑦Any diameter of the diagram can divide it into two semicircles. The areas of yin and yang in a semicircle is mostly unequal except special condition. It indicates that in concrete matters, yin and yang are always imbalanced; but on the whole, they are balanced. The overall balance is based on the concrete imbalance.

⑧Any diameter through the center of Tai ji diagram divides it into two semicircles. Any semicircle contains yin and yang. It shows any thing or phenomenon consists of yin and yang. Nothing is composed purely of yin or yang.

⑨A Tai ji diagram can be considered to be composed of innumerable little Tai ji diagrams. The yin-yang growth and decline of Tai ji diagram is resulted from the yin-yang transformation of these tiny diagrams. While the yin-yang transformation of Tai ji diagram itself occurs when its yin-yang growth and decline develops to extremity. Therefore, yin-yang transformation is the consequence of yin-yang growth and decline on the same level, and yin-yang growth and decline is consequence of yin-yang transformation on the lower level. It indicates that yin-yang transformation and yin-yang growth and decline are mutual rooting and restriction.

3. Application of yin-yang theory on medicine

Yin-yang theory is the guiding ideology and methodology of TCM theory. It is throughout every aspect of TCM. Relation of man and nature, physiological, pathological, pharmacological effects, clinical diagnosis and treatment, and so on, have to be analyzed and handled with the guidance and methods of yin-yang theory.

(1) To materialize the relation of man and nature

There is yin-yang in heaven and earth and even the human body. They correspond with each other. It provides theoretical bases for integrity and correspondence of man and universe.

Yang rises in spring and summer and falls in autumn and winter, which is the yin-yang growth and decline in four seasons. In nature, it causes sprout in spring, growth in summer, harvest in autumn and store in winter, and it is same in the human body, based on which the thought of nourishing yang in spring and summer and tonifying yin in autumn and winter is raised.

In one day, yang is born from 11:00 pm to 1:00 am, and grows to extreme at noon. Yin is born from 1:00 pm to 3:00 pm, and grows to extreme from 9:00 pm to 11:00 pm. The rise and fall of yin-yang will cause correspondent changes in human bodies, which provides theoretical bases for clinical diagnosis, circulation of channel qi and opening and closing of acupoint as well as the clinical estimate of yin-yang excess and deficiency and timely acupoint selection of acupuncture.

(2) Establishment of demic physiological theory

①The analysis of yin-yang attributes of demic structure. The analysis is generally based on up and down, inside and outside, and so on. Taking the human body as a example, the part above waist is yang and the part below is yin; the surface of the body is yang and inner parts are yin; six fu-organs are yang and five internal organs are yin; in the five internal organs, lung and heart are yang, liver, spleen and kidney are yin. The part above waist is yang, so it is often hit by wind-heat and yang evil; the part below waist is yin, so it is mostly hit by cold-dampness and yin evil. The surface is yang, so the six evils always hit it from the outside; the inner parts are yin, so evils of food, fatigue and seven human emotions hit them from inside. Six fu-organs are yang, whose functions are mainly transportation and transformation to ensure the body is unobstructed, so diseases of six fu-organs are often heat or excess syndrome; five internal organs are yin, and their function is mainly to store vital essence, so diseases of the five internal organs are cold or deficiency syndrome. Heart and lung are yang. One belongs to fire and another governs qi, and they together govern qi and blood, so diseases about heart and lung are manifested as yang-heat syndrome; liver, spleen and kidney are yin, and they govern essence and blood, so their diseases are mostly deficiency or cold.

Due to different yin-yang attributes of the demic structure, they are physiologically and pathologically different, and provide bases for clinical diagnosis and treatment.

②Establishing physiological theory. Combined with specific conditions, it is established under the guidance of yin-yang theory.

The physiological theory based on yin-yang theory adopts dichotomy; among the viscera of the human body, internal organs are yin which governs store and fu-organs are yang governing transformation; in terms of every viscus, each has yin-yang and qi and blood. Yin blood dominates nourishing and moistening, and yang qi dominates warming and arousing; in terms of the whole, except yin-yang, qi and blood, there are ying-wei and fluid. These are representation of dichotomy. Therefore, they are opposite and complementary and considered as pairs of yin and yang to fulfill their physiological functions.

The qi transformation refers to the transformation of matters and energy inside the body. It happens during the ascending, descending, exiting and entering of qi. In *Su Wen · Liu Wei Zhi Da Lun*, it writes that "qi's ascending and descending are the consequence of heaven-earth reaction ... Heaven's qi descends and flows to earth; earth's qi ascends and flies in heaven. It is because qi of heaven and earth join together that everything changes and life is created and maintained. " Actually, the interaction of qi in heaven and earth is actually that of yin qi and yang qi. Therefore, qi transformation is caused by yin-yang ascending and descending. In terms of the human body, ascending and descending are qi's motion inside, and exiting and entering are exchange materials with the outside. In *Su Wen · Liu Wei Zhi Da Lun*, it says that if exiting and entering stop, the human body will no longer exchange materials with the outside, and then life cannot be maintained; if ascending and descending stop, qi will no longer exist. It indicates the importance of qi's motion and transformation in the life. Actually, it is the concrete explanation of yin-yang theory to vital phenomena.

Yin-yang balance, yin-yang growth and decline and yin-yang transformation are all basic viewpoints of the TCM physiology.

(3) Establishment of pathological theory

① Understanding of pathogenesis. In *Internal Classic*, yin-yang has been used to learn pathogenic factors. It suggests that pathogenic factors from climatic changes, such as wind, rain, cold and heat invade from skin, and come to viscera through meridians and collaterals; others like mental and diet factors hurt viscera internally. Therefore, in *Su Wen · Tiao Jing Lun*, it says: "Evils are born of yin or yang. Yang evils are from wind, rain, cold and heat; yin evils are from diet, shelter, yin, yang, joy and anger. In *Internal Classic*, wind, rain, cold and dampness are categorized into yin-yang in light of their attributes. Wind and rain transformed from qi of heaven result in excess syndromes; cold and dampness transformed from qi of earth result in deficiency syndromes. "

② Establishment of pathological theory. Yin-yang balance and coordination are the bases of TCM physiological theory, prerequisites to maintain man's normal physiological functions. While yin-yang imbalance is the foot stone of TCM pathology.

Yin-yang imbalance is, on the one hand, caused by exogenous evils that destroy the balance, and on the other hand, caused by the viscera maladjustment.

External evils can be divided according to yin-yang. When act on human body, they can cause excess or deficiency of yin-yang. In *Su Wen · Yin-yang Ying Xiang Da Lun*, it writes: "Excess of yin causes yang diseases, and excess of yang causes yin diseases. Excess of yang leads to heat and excess of yin leads to cold. " These are presentation of yin-yang maladjustment due to exogenous evils. Yang diseases and cold syndromes are often caused by exogenous yin evil, which gives rise to excess of yin-cold, deficiency of yang qi. yang qi's warming function gets disordered, so the cold symptoms appear. Yin diseases and heat often occur as the result of exogenous warmth and heat, which results in excess of yang qi and wastage of yin qi. Because yin qi cannot restrict yang, so appears heat symptoms. With regard to symptoms of yin-yang excess caused by exogenous evils, the excessive side is dominant, while the deficient one is relative, so this kind of diseases are mostly excess symptoms.

Viscera maladjustment is often caused by seven emotions, diet, fatigue, excessive sexual intercourse, and so on. It directly acts on viscera, causes disorder in yin-yang and qi and blood, and leads to their deficiency. Deficiency of yin corresponds to excess of yang which gives rise to deficiency fever, so it leads to heat. Deficiency of yang corresponds to excess of yin which gives rise to deficiency cold, so it leads to cold.

Due to yin-yang rooting, yin and yang can mutually generate each other. Therefore, when yin or yang cannot generate the other because of extreme deficiency, it will necessarily involve the opposite side and lead to deficiency of the both sides. This is the pathological process that impairment of yin involves yang and the vise versa.

Diseases can obstruct the yin-yang restriction and lead to abnormal yin-yang growth and decline, which worsens yin-yang maladjustment. When yin-yang grows or declines to a extreme level, it can

192

transform. In *Su Wen · Yin-yang Ying Xiang Da Lun*, it says: "Extreme cold causes heat and extreme heat causes cold", and "Extreme yin generates yang and extreme yang generates yin". These are all resulted from yin-yang transformation. However, heat developing to cold and excess symptoms developing to deficiency ones are consequences of disease progression. While cold syndromes with heat manifestation and deficiency syndromes with excess manifestation are all false appearance instead of improvement. In short, these occur when the condition gets serious.

(4) Application on clinical diagnosis

The occurrence of diseases is always resulted from yin-yang maladjustment, so it seems important to distinguish yin and yang during diagnosis. In *Su Wen · Yin-yang Ying Xiang Da Lun*, it says that a good diagnostician first observes complexion and takes the pulse to distinguish yin and yang.

To distinguish yin and yang has two implications: one is to distinguish the yin-yang attributes of symptoms; the other is to distinguish yin symptoms and yang symptoms.

To distinguish yin-yang attributes is one mission of the four methods of diagnosis. The first one is to distinguish according to shade of colors. The bright are in yang fen and belong to excess and heat symptoms; the dark are in yin fen and belong to deficiency and cold symptoms. The second one is to distinguish from voices. The loud and loquacious are mostly excess and heat symptoms; the low and silent are mostly deficiency and cold symptoms. The third one is to distinguish from pulse conditions. The floating, large, rapid and full pulses are yang; the deep, thready, retarded and weak pulses are yin. To distinguish by the four methods of diagnosis provides bases for the differentiation of yin and yang symptoms.

At first, the differentiation should be carried out according to the eight principals, i. e. , exterior and interior, deficiency and excess, chills and fever and yin and yang among which yin and yang are the general principle, exterior and interior are to distinguish disease location, chills and fever are to distinguish the attributes of disease, and deficiency and excess are to distinguish the mutual condition of evil and health. The disease location is either exterior or interior; the attributes are cold, heat, dry or damp; the mutual condition of evil and health is either deficiency or excess. After those above have been distinguished, it can be inferred that exterior, heat and excess syndromes are yang; interior, cold and deficiency syndromes are yin.

(5) To guide clinical treatment

In *Su Wen · Yin Yang Ying Xiang Da Lun*, it says that to regulate yin-yang according to diagnosis, the aim is to enable it to get back to balance. It indicates that to regulate yin-yang and get it back to balance are the basic principles of TCM treatment.

The methods of conditioning yin-yang are on the basis of its excess and deficiency. It is wise to dispel the excess and complement the deficiency. If it is excess, then effuse it; if it is deficiency, then complement it.

To the yin-yang excess, the extra part should be dispelled. Ex-

194

cess of yang gives rise to heat, so it should be weakened by cold medicines. Excess of yin generates cold, so it should be impaired by warm medicines. To yin-yang deficiency, it should be treated through complementary. Deficiency of yang leads to cold, so yang qi should be complemented by warm tonics. Deficiency of yin causes heat, so sweet-cold tonics ought to be applied to nourish yin and expel extra heat.

When condition and nourish yin-yang, it is necessary to pay attention to the principles of yin-yang mutual rooting. Zhang Jingyue said: " To complement yang, yin tonics must be added at the same time; to complement yin, yang tonics must be added, thus yin and yang can mutually transform. "

Part Ⅱ Five-element Theory

Same with yin-yang theory, five-element theory is the philosophy of Chinese ancient naive materialism and dialectics and once took important position in history.

1. The formation of five-element concepts

The concept of five elements was formed very early. It has appeared at least since Shang and Zhou Dynasties.

It was formed in the ancients' life. They found that wood, fire, earth, metal and water are five indispensable matters of people's life, thus comes out the concept of five materials. In *Zuo Zhuan*, it says: "Nature generates the five materials. People use them all and no one can be omitted. " It is also said in *Shang Shu*: "Water and fire are necessary for diet; metal and wood are necessary for labor; earth is what everything in nature relies on. " Five materials are proposed from the point of people's necessity in life, so they are indispensable.

Wood, fire, earth, metal and water are necessary in man's life, and the daily supplies are made of them. For example, the earthen jar is made from earth and water and then fired; houses are built by wood, earth and water; the tools for hunting and farming are made from wood and metal. According to these examples, the ancients further imagined that everything in nature also consists of these five mat-

196

ters. Just as it is said in *Guo Yu*, sages mixed earth with metal, wood, water and fire to make various things. "Thus, wood, fire, earth, metal and water were considered as the elements that made up everything in nature, which obviously does not make sense. If replace the the concrete matters with abstract attributes, it seems more reasonable. Hence, in *Shang Shu · Hong Fan*, it says that water is to nourish and flow downwards, fire is to warm and ascend, wood is to grow in either a bent or straight way, metal is easy to transform, and earth is able to grow crops. " To abstract the features of the five concrete matters as the connotation of wood, fire, earth, metal and water enables the five elements to change from concrete matters to abstract concepts that only represent these five attributes.

Till that time, the philosophical five-element concepts were preliminarily formed. It holds that any thing or phenomenon in the world contains the five attributes——wood, fire, earth, metal and water, and the mutual relations of them determine the occurrence and development; the differences between things or phenomena are stipulated by the moving conditions of the five attributes.

In the end of the Warring States Period, by inference of five elements, essence theory, yin-yang theory and five-element theory were blended together, Zou Yan established the yin-yang and five-element theory and further perfected five-element theory.

2. The basic contents of five-element theory

The basic contents of five-element theory include five-element classification, five-element generation, restriction, supervision and transformation, and five-element invasion and insult.

(1) Five-element classification

Based on attributes of the five elements, the classification makes analogy between things or phenomena and one attribute, and then five big systems are formed.

The attributes that five elements represent are abstracted from concrete wood, fire, earth, metal and water.

Features of wood: including all grass and trees, the growing characteristics of wood is that their limbs are bent or straight and they stretch upward or outward to the best so as to strive for more sunshine and better living condition; the branches are soft, easy to bend and recover; they have strong vitality, and as long as the condition is satisfying, they can live stubbornly. The ancients summarized the characteristics of wood as germination, soft, bent and straight, stretching, and so on.

Features of fire: fire is warm, bright with upward flame. It leads the air to flow upwards. The ancients summarized its features as upward flame, yang heat, rising, and so on.

Features of earth: earth bears everything and everything comes from it, which proves that what in earth is essential for the growth of everything. Everything in nature is buried in earth. It can be rotted and then disappear. The ancients generalized its features as growth and nourishment, generation and transformation, receiving, changing, and so on.

Features of metal: the earliest metal that humans found is tin and then copper. Considering the color of tin, they think that metal is white. The features of metal are: firstly, it has good heat conductivity, so people feel it cool; secondly, it is not easily contaminated, and despite of being contaminated, it can be easily washed off; thirdly, it has large specific gravity, so people feel it heavy; fourthly metal is rigid and ductile; fifthly, it can be melted by fire and cast arbitrarily. The ancients summarized its features as cool, clean, purification and descending, astringency, and so on.

Features of water: water is fluid, flows downwards and can wet things. Water is cold and able to put out fire. Even if in hot summer, water in the well is still freezing cold. The ancients generalized the features as cold and damp, flowing downwards, moistening, and so on.

The five-element theory holds that the universe consists of matters with attributes of wood, fire, earth, metal and water. Therefore, any thing or phenomenon can be categorized according to five elements. For example, a year can be divided into five seasons——spring, summer, late summer, autumn and winter; climates can be classified as five qi—— wind, summer heat, dampness, dryness and cold; directions can be classified as east, south, middle, west and north; colors can be classified into green, red, yellow, white and black; creatures' vital process can be divided into five transformations——germination, growth, transformation, harvest and storing; flavors can be divided into sour, bitter, sweet, pungent and salty; a day can be divided into daybreak, noon, sundown, evening and midnight; in the human body there are five internal organs—— liver, heart, spleen, lung and kidney, five fu-organs——gallbladder, small intestine, stomach, large intestine and bladder, five body constituents——tendons, vessel, muscle, hair and bones, five sense organs——eyes, tongue, mouth, nose and ears, five mentations—— soul, mind, intention, vigor and will, and five emotions——anger, joy, thought, sadness and fear.

Five seasons, five qi, five transformations, five internal organs and five sense organs all can be categorized into five elements according to analogy of attributes. For example, wood is featured with germination, while in spring plants sprout, it is the beginning of growth circle and full of vigor, so spring falls into category of wood; while spring also means the ground turning green, so green also belongs to wood; the east of China is coast with favorable climatic weathers for plants' growth, so east belongs to wood; germination is the beginning of life circle, so it belongs to wood; before fruits are ripe, they are usually sour, so sour belongs to wood; daybreak is the start of a day and when sun rises from the east, yang qi begins to ascend, so daybreak belongs to wood. Through inference and analogy like this, spring, wind, green, east, birth, sour, daybreak and so on, are all categorized in wood. Applied on the human body, liver's function is to distribute qi's activity and in favor of free flow, so it belongs to wood; gallbladder and liver are relation of exterior and interior, and gallbladder is attached to liver; liver dominates tendons which rely on nourishment of liver; liver resuscitates at eyes, harmonious liver qi helps eyes distinguish black and white; soul hides in liver; liver controls

200

anger. Therefore, in the human body, liver, gallbladder, tendons, eyes, soul and anger are categorized in wood.

Table of Five-element Classification

Elements	Attributes	Seasons	Directions	Transformation	Colors	Flavors	Qi
Wood	germination streching	spring	east	germination	green	sour	wind
Fire	hot, upward flame	summer	south	growth	red	bitter	Summer heat
Earth	growth, nourishment, transformation	late summer	middle	alteration	yellow	sweet	dampness
Metal	purification, descending, astringency	autumn	west	reaping	white	pungent	dryness
Water	cold, damp, flowing downward	winter	north	storing	black	salty	cold

Elements	Times	Tones	Cereals	Livestock	Internal organs	Fu-organs	Body constituent
Wood	daybreak	jiao	fiber	dog	liver	gallbladder	tendon
Fire	noon	zheng	wheat	horse	heart	small intestine	vessel
Earth	sundown	gong	millet	cattle	spleen	stomach	muscle
Metal	evening	shang	rice	chicken	lung	large intestine	hair
Water	midnight	yu	beans	pig	kidney	bladder	bones

For either nature or human, the premise that they can be classified according to attributes of five elements lies on integrity of nature and human, and seasons, directions, climates, vital process, colors, day and night, flavors, or organs, entrails, shapes, sense organs, mentations and emotions mentioned above can separately become a relatively independent whole. Five-element classification is only appropriate for analysis and classification of the relatively independent whole.

(2) Five-element generation, restriction, supervision and transformation

Five-element theory is not only a classification, but also a theory that can clarify the general rule of things' interior movements. Things are always separable and constituted by several parts. The constituents connect with each other in some ways and move endlessly. Five-element theory is to use generation and restriction to clarify the balance and coordination of every constituent, i. e. , the concrete way that how things maintain their integrity, unity and stability.

The ancients summarized the ways that things connect as mutual benefit and mutual damage. In five-element theory, mutual benefit is called mutual generation, and mutual damage as mutual restriction. Mutual generation means mutual support, nourishment and reinforcement between things; mutual restriction means mutual inhibition, opposition, fight and control between them. Five-element theory use mutual generation and restriction to illustrate the connecting ways of five elements and the mechanism of maintaining balance and coordina-

202

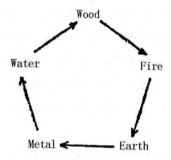

Figure 8. **Five – element generation**

tion inside things or phenomena.

The mutual generation and restriction can be normal or abnormal. Five-element theory calls abnormal generation and restriction as invasion and insult.

①Five-element generation and restriction. It means that between five elements, they mutually generate and restrict each other in a normal way.

Mutual generation of five elements has its sequence: wood generates fire, fire generates earth, earth generates metal and metal generates water. The sequence was worked out according observation to natural phenomena. For example, fire can be made by drilling wood and twigs can be lighted by fire, so it is thought that wood can generate fire; burned-out things become ashes which are earth, so fire can generate earth; metal is extracted from minerals which are mined from beneath the earth, and the ancients thought the minerals were made from earth, so earth can generate metal; vapor is easily to condense to water, and where there are many mountains there is plenty vapor. On mountains there must be stones in which contains a lot of metal. In damp and moist caves, there always will be dropping water or gushing spring. The ancients thought the water qi is transformed from metal qi, so metal generates water. Though plants root from earth, they cannot grow on land without water, so it was thought that water can generate wood.

In *Difficult Classic*, the mutual generation of five elements is called mother-child relation. The generating one is mother and the generated is the child. In terms of water generating wood, water is mother of wood; wood generates fire, so fire is son of wood.

Mutual generation of five elements also develops in certain sequence. One restricts the next but one. Given the sequence of wood, fire, earth, metal and water, wood restricts earth, earth restricts wa-

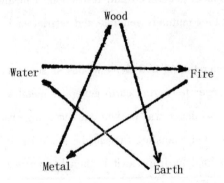

Figure 9. Five – element restriction

ter, water restricts fire, fire restricts metal and metal restricts wood. The sequence of five-element restriction is generalized from the observation of natural phenomena. No matter how hard the earth is, plants are always able to break through, and then soil becomes spongy. The plants' roots are soft and thin, they cannot be obstructed by the hardest earth, so it is said that wood can restrict earth; earth can block water, and after a water hole is filled up by earth, water is dried, so earth can restrict water; water can put out fire, so water restricts fire; fire can melt metal, so fire restricts metal; metal cutters can be used for woodcutting, so metal restricts wood. The five-element restriction is described in *Su Wen · Bao Ming Quan Xing Lun*.

In *Internal Classic*, the restrictive relation of five elements is described as relation of inheritance and supervision. For example, in *Su Wen · Liu Wei Zhi Da Lun*, it is said that ministerial fire is followed by water qi; beneath water level, it is inherited by earth qi. In *Internal Classic*, the mutual restriction is also called mutual conquering which means that addition is bound to win. For example of one specific element, the elements restricted by it is called "conquered", and those restricting it is called "conquerer". Taking wood for example, metal restricts wood, and then wood cannot conquer metal, and metal is conquerer of wood; wood restricts earth, so wood can conquer earth, and earth is the conquered of wood.

Among the mutual relations of five elements, every element will connect the others in the way of either generation or restriction. There are two kinds of generation——"generator" and "generated", so is restriction——restricter and restricted. Taking wood for example, wood connects water and fire in the way of generation, i. e. , water generates wood which generates fire, so in terms of wood, water is

205

"generator" of wood and fire is "generated" of wood; wood is in restrictive relation with metal and fire, i. e. , metal restricts wood which restricts earth, so in terms of wood, metal is "restricter" of wood, and earth is "restricted" of wood.

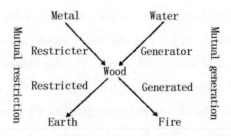

Figure 10.　**The relationships of restriction and generation between wood and other four elements**

Every element relates the other four in the way of generation or restriction. It is not only restricted by the others, but also restricts them. Thus, they form mutual dependent and restrictive relation, through which they maintain balance and coordination and form an organic whole. Therefore, every element cannot separate from the others to exist independently. Any change of an element will affect and be affected by the others. It is because of this that five elements become a rather strict and stable structure.

②Five-element invasion and insult. They are abnormal connections between five elements and caused by abnormal quantity of five elements or excessive restriction.

Invasion is expression of excessive restriction. Insult is mainly reverse restriction.

206

The causes of five-element invasion and insult are two: one is because the element exceeds the permitted fluctuation range of five-element balance, which gives rise to abnormal excess. The consequence of abnormal excess is bound to excessively restrict the "restricted", i. e. , invasion. At the same time, it reversely restricts the "restricter", i. e. , insult. The other is because the element is overly weak and also exceeds the permitted fluctuation range, which leads to abnormal insufficiency. Abnormal insufficiency makes the element unable to restrict the others and reversely restricted by them, i. e. insult. Relative excessive restriction emerges because another element that restricts it is abnormally insufficient, i. e. invasion. In *Su Wen · Wu Xing Yun Da Lun*, it says that if qi is excessive, then the "conquered" is overly restricted and the "conquerer" is insulted; if qi is insufficient, then the "conquerer" is insulted by its "conquered" and invaded by its "conquerer", and the "conquered" easily insults its "conquerer".

Five-element invasion is the phenomenon that restriction exceeds normal range, but it is still in normal restriction direction. Therefore, the direction of five-element invasion and restriction is consistent, i. e. , wood invades earth, earth invades water, water invades fire, fire invades metal and metal invades wood.

Mutual invasion is excess of restriction, so clinically it is called restriction. For example, wood invades earth, clinically it is called wood restricts earth; water invades fire, and clinically it is called water qi attacking heart. It is because what is revolved clinically are mostly pathogenic phenomena instead of physiological restric-

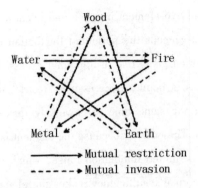

Figure 11.　Five – element invasion

tion. Pathogenic restriction is invasion, and pure physiological restriction is not invasion.

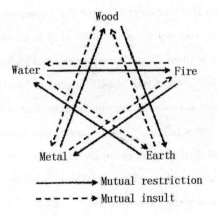

Figure 12.　Five – element insult

Five-element insult is due to five-element rise and fall exceeding normal permitted range which causes abnormal restriction. It may be abnormal on the intensity of restriction, but it is mainly on the direction of restriction, i. e. , reverse restriction. That is, it is opposite to normal restriction of five elements, so it is also called reverse restriction. The sequence of five-element insult is that wood insults metal, metal insults fire, fire insults water, water insults earth and earth insults wood.

On clinic, the name of insult is not consistent. For example, earth insults wood, and it is called obstruction of earth and depression of wood; wood insults metal, and it is called wood-fire impairing metal; others like heart fire burning kidney yin is manifestation of fire insulting water, and lung heat transmitting to heart is pathogenic manifestation of metal insulting fire.

③ Five-element generation and restriction. Between five elements, there are two connecting ways: generation and restriction. It maintains balance and coordination inside things, further preserves stability, unity, integrity and their normal movement, i. e. , things' normal vital process. The supervision between things' constituent parts maintains the balance and coordination, so does the stability, unity and integrity. Transformation happens under the condition of interior unity, coordination and balance.

In *Su Wen · Liu Wei Zhi Da Lun*, it says that excess leads to abnormality, and inheritance leads to supervision. Supervision promotes generation and transformation which externally is manifested as normal vital process with rise and fall; abnormality gives rise to destruction of interior balance and coordination, and serious disorder of generation and transformation will threaten the life and existence of things. It indicates that the five-element generation, restriction, supervision and transformation maintain the existence and normal vital movement of five elements.

In *Lei Jing Tu Yi*, by Zhang Jingyue of the Ming Dynasty, it says that all creatures and their movements cannot be without generation as well as restriction. No generation, no source of growth; no restriction, there will be excess or deficiency. Therefore, Zhang Jingyue also thought that generation, restriction, supervision and transformation between five elements are the fundamental reasons to maintain things' existence as well as their vital generation and development.

About the specific methods of five-element generation, restriction, supervision and transformation, in *Su Wen · Zhi Zhen Yao Da Lun*, it is written that: "Conquer causes transformation, transformation gives rise to conquer, and without transformation is dangerous." It means that when the restrictive power between things reaches to the maximum, they will transform into the opposite sides; when the restrictive power declines to the minimum, things will transform in the direction that restriction is enhanced. Without alternation of rise and fall, it will ruin the normal relation between things. In *Su Wen · Tian Yuan Ji Da Lun*, it says: "The process of five-element rise and fall is the consequence of their coordination and restriction, and each one goes through the course of excess and deficiency. Therefore, at the beginning, with the gradual disappear of excess, the deficiency comes, and the vice versa." In other words, during the process of things' existence, generation and development, they always present the alternation of excess and deficiency, which is resulted from five-element regulation function. It turns out that any thing or phenomenon's process of existence, generation and development is not static or balanced. It is dynamic and achieved in the course of imbalance and movement so as to maintain stability and existence.

Each element has its own rise and fall, which gives rise to correspondent change of mutual generation and restriction. Mutual generation and restriction are to maintain balance and coordination between five elements. Therefore, under normal circumstances, the force of mutual generation is in direct proportion to the element's rise and fall, and the force of mutual restriction is in inverse direction to it. The relation between five-element rise and fall and its generation and restriction not only maintain the existence, what more important is that it maintains balance and coordination between five elements, as well as their unity, integrity and stability. For example, in the world of animals, herbivores are lack of defense ability, but they are more fertile and live in large groups made up by tens or hundreds of them; aggressive predators are less fertile and live in small groups. Therefore, herbivores have advantages in quantity due to higher reproductive capacity, which not only satisfies predators's need for food (mutual generation), but also ensures species reproduction; though predators' reproductive capacity is weak and they are disadvantaged in quantity, they attacks fiercely with high probability (mutual restriction), so they can capture enough food to ensure the species reproduction. Herbivores' advantage in quantity (self-prosperity themselves) ensures predators' food supply (mutual generation is relatively strong), but they are not strong enough to defend themselves against predators (mutual restriction is weak); predators' weakness in quantity (self-weakness) determines that they are insufficient to support other creatures (mutual generation is weak), while they are strong in both attack and defense (mutual restriction is strong). Herbivores, predators and other creatures are different in quantity, supporting other species, self-defense ability, and so on, which helps them survive, reproduce and preserve ecological balance, and guarantees natural prosperity. It is the result of natural selection.

When five-element restriction is in direct proportion to an element's rise and fall, it will necessarily drive the rising one stronger and the falling one weaker, and finally lead to destruction of balance and coordination as well as disappearance of five-element unity, integrity, stability, and even the things existing as a whole. As a result, under this circumstance, it becomes a destroying factor, which belongs to abnormal condition of five-element restriction.

In order to illustrate how five elements keep balance and coordination through "generation and restriction", Zhang Jingyue proposed the specific ways of five-element generation, restriction, supervision and transformation, i. e. ,five-element conquer and revenge.

In *Lei Jing Tu Yi*, it says that in terms of five-element conquer and revenge, where there is conquer, there is defeat; there is defeat and there will be revenge; "mother" is defeated, and "child" will inevitably save her. For example, excess of water hurts fire, and earth, child of fire, will necessarily restrict it. . . In other words, excess of water qi leads to abnormal restriction (restrictive is in direct ratio to rise and fall). Water's over-restriction to fire hurts fire qi, which results in fire's inability to give birth to earth——decline of earth. Under normal circumstances, the restrictive power is in inverse proportion to an element's rise and fall, so earth qi strengthens restriction to water qi, which enables water qi to recover; water's restriction to fire is weaker, and fire qi recovers; the function that fire generates earth becomes stronger, and earth qi recovers; the power that earth restricts water weakens, and the three elements come back to normal condition.

In the examples above, water's restriction to fire is abnormal, i. e. , pathological restriction, so the power that water restricts fire is in direct proportion to water's rise and fall; while earth's restriction to eat is normal, i. e. , physiological restriction, so the power that earth restricts water is in inverse proportion to earth's rise and fall. They are different.

Besides, only water, fire and earth are mentioned. While in fact, metal and wood also take part in the regulation. Water rises, and the function that water generates wood strengthens; if wood qi is vigorous, then the function that wood generates fire strengthens, which is useful to resist water's restriction to fire in case of deficiency of fire qi and excess of wood qi, and the function that wood restricts wood weakens, it avoids deficiency of wood qi. Restricted by water, fire declines, while the function that fire restricts metal strengthens; deficient fire

213

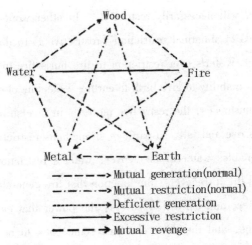

Figure 13.　Five - element conquer and revenge

cannot generate earth, and declining earth cannot generate metal. All is to weaken metal qi, so it cannot generate water. Therefore, except water, fire and metal, between wood metal also exists correspondent generation and restriction, which aims to prevent fire and wood from over-declining and restrict excess of water, so as to quickly restore five-element balance and coordination that already lost.

It is through generation, restriction, supervision and transformation that five elements maintain balance and coordination and preserve unity, integrity, stability and further existence of matters.

④Dialectical relation of five-element generation and restriction. It is mainly manifested in two aspects: one is its relation with quantity; the other is mutual-use relation between generation and restriction, i. e. , there is generation in restriction and restriction in generation.

The first aspect means that five-element generation and restriction have something to do with the proportion of each element's quantity. The rules of five-element generation and restriction mentioned above are mainly in terms of average constant, i. e. , variation of each element's growth and decline which are limited within permitted fluctuation range of balance and coordination. Only on this condition can those rules be established. If conditions vary, when five-element growth and decline exceed the permitted fluctuation range, especially the proportion of growth and decline, then the rules cannot exist.

For example, water generates wood, which is based on right proportion of water and wood's growth and decline. When water is adequate, wood grows prosperously. If the proportion is not appropriate, insufficient water cannot solve drought that has already happened, so even if there is water again, plants cannot sprout; excessive water leads to flood which kills wood. Wood can generate fire when proportion of them is rational. If throw a huge wood on fire, fire will not become bigger but be put out. Therefore, the proportion of "mother" and "child" has to be matched. That is, their quantity must be limited within a permitted fluctuation range of balance, and the mutual generation happens; if the proportion is not matched and exceeds the permitted range, then the relation that "mother generates child" will be destroyed, i. e. , "strong mother" cannot generate "weak child", or "weak mother" cannot generate "strong child".

Five-element restriction also must be limited within the range of constant. If it exceeds the permitted range, then the rules of restriction cannot be established. Earth restricts water only on the condition that they are both in right proportion, thus earth can prevent flood. Water

215

restricts fire, but if a glass of water is used for putting out raging flame, fire will not die out but be made bigger. It proves that during mutual restriction, it is necessary for the restricting and restricted sides to be equivalent in quantity. If not, the restrictive relation will be changed.

Therefore, in the relation of five-element generation and restriction exists quantitative relation. Only when generation and restriction are equivalent can they be in sequence; if not, the sequence will vanish. It is the meaning of "five elements are not ever-victorious" and "five elements inversely generate and restrict each other".

Only when five-element generation and restriction are within a constant range can the sequence be established, which refers to the proportional relation of five-element rise and fall. The proportional relation actually means five-element rise-fall fluctuation. It can only be limited within the permitted fluctuation range of five-element balance and coordination. This is normal fluctuation. Once exceeds the range, it is abnormal and will inevitably cause abnormal restriction, i. e. , five-element invasion and insult.

The mutual use of five-element generation and restriction refers to "restriction in generation" and "use in restriction" proposed by Zhang Jingyue. In *Lei Jing Tu Yi*, it says that people only know five-element generation but do not realize that restriction is included during the process; they only know five-element restriction but do not know that the aim of restriction is to enable the restricted function normally. Zhang Jingyue realized that mutual restriction and destruction exist in mutual generation, while the target of mutual restriction is mutual

216

use. For the example of wood generating fire, wood is burned by fire and finally disappear; for the example of fire generating earth, things are burned into ashes which belong to earth, if ashes accumulate too much, fire will be covered by them and cannot grow bigger. Wood helps fire burn stronger, while itself is harmed by fire; fire increases the quantity of earth, while it will take away the flames. The consequence of five-element generation is that "child" is born while "mother" is harmed. Therefore, five-element generation contains mutual restriction and destruction, i. e. ,the phenomenon of "child" restricting or hurting "mother".

Five-element restriction is to enable the "restricted" function normally. For example, if fire is restricted by water, it will lead to coordination of water and fire, which controls fire within permitted range and activates the warming function. If water cannot restrict fire, the latter will be excessively hot and finally burn down everything. Earth restricts water within normal range, so water is capable of moistening and coordinating itself with fire. If earth cannot restrict water, water qi will be out of control and causes disaster. Therefore, the objective of five-element restriction is to control the "restricted" and make them function normally.

What is said above illustrates that the essence of five-element generation is transformation, i. e. ,to transform "mother" to "child"; the essence of five-element restriction is to make the "restricted" function normally, containing mutual generation and mutual use. Mutual generation and restriction are both opposite and complementary to each other, and they are dialectical.

3. Medical application of five-element theory

(1) Expression of man-nature unity

Five-element theory classifies structure and function of the human body into five elements, as well as five seasons, five directions, five times, five qi, five flavors, five colors, and so on. Through five elements, nature and human bodies are unified together and become a unity, which concretely explains the theories——"unity of man and nature" and "correspondence between man and universe", and provides theoretical bases for holism of TCM. Five sense organs——eyes, tongue, mouth, nose and ears, five mentations——soul, mind, intention, vigor and will, and five emotions——anger, joy, miss, sadness and fear.

Table of Man-nature Unity

Nature							Five elements and Attributes
Seasons	Directions	Changes	Colors	Flavors	Climates	Times	
spring	east	germination	green	sour	wind	daybreak	Wood (germination, stretching)
summer	south	growth	red	bitter	Summer heat	noon	Fire (hot, upward flame)
late summer	middle	alteration	yellow	sweet	dampness	sundown	Earth (growth, nourishment, transformation)
autumn	west	reaping	white	pungent	dryness	evening	Metal (purification, descending, astringency)
winter	north	storing	black	salty	cold	midnight	Water (cold, damp, flowing downwards)

218

Human body					
Internal organs	Fu-organs	Body con-stituents	Sense organs	Mentations	Emotions
liver	gallbladder	tendons	eyes	soul	anger
heart	small intestine	vessel	tongue	mind	joy
spleen	stomach	muscle	mouth	intention	thought
lung	large intestine	hair	nose	vigor	sadness
kidney	bladder	bones	ears	will	fear

Through five elements, the human body and nature are unified. For example, the connection between five internal organs and seasons: liver qi abounds in spring, heart qi in summer, spleen qi in autumn, kidney qi in winter; diseases of liver are prone to occur in autumn, diseases of heart are in winter, diseases of spleen are in spring, diseases of lung are in summer, diseases of kidney are in late summer. The connection between five internal organs and five qi: wind impairs liver, summer heat impairs heart, dampness impairs spleen, dryness impairs lung, cold impairs hurts kidney. Every kind of phenomenon in nature can be related with human body by the connection so as to explain the content of correspondence between man and universe.

(2) Establishing the demic physiological theory

① Clarifying physiological functions of five internal organs through the attributes of five elements. Five-element theory categorizes five internal organs into five elements, and applies five-element attributes to clarify the physiological functions of internal organs'. Wood is

219

bent or straight, inclines to stretch and has the feature of germination; liver communicates with wood-qi, so liver inclines to spread out freely and governs catharsis and ascending. Fire is warm and flames are upward; heart communicates with fire-qi, so it governs warming and circulation of blood so as to warm and nourish the whole body. Earth is thick and solid, which grows and transforms everything, so it governs growth and transformation; spleen communicates with earth-qi, governing transportation and transformation of essence of water and grain, so it is the foundation of acquired constitution and the source of growth and transformation. Metal is cool and clean, governing purification, descending and astringency; lung communicates with metal-qi, governing breathing, managing exchange of the pure and the turbid. And the lung-qi governs purification and descending and circulates water. Water is cold, mildly laxative, governing hiding and storing; kidney communicates with water-qi, so it governs storing, mainly storing up essence and being in charge of qi transformation of watery fluid. To explain five internal organs' physiological function by means of five elements is an important aspect of the application of five-element theory in medicine.

Table of Five-element Attributes and the Physiological Functions of Five Internal Organs

Elements	Attributes	Internal organs	Functions
Wood	germination stretching	liver	spread out freely, governs catharsis, ascending
Fire	hot, upward flame	heart	governs warming and circulation of blood, warm and nourish the whole body
Earth	growth, nourishment, transformation	spleen	governs transportation and transformation of essence of water and grain, source of growth and transformation
Metal	purification, descending, astringency	lung	governs breathing, manages exchange of the pure and the turbid, purifies and descends, circulates water
Water	cold, damp, flowing downward	kidney	governs storing, mainly storing up essence and being in charge of qi transformation of watery fluid

②Clarifying five internal organs' relation with five-element generation, restriction, supervision and transformation. Five-element theory takes use of five-element generation, restriction, supervision and transformation to explain the physiological relation between five internal organs, which helps to organize them into an organic whole. To clarify the mechanism that preserves balance and coordination inside human bodies with mutual help and restriction between five internal organs provides theoretical bases to prove that human being is a organic whole.

Clarifying mutual-help relation between five internal organs with five-element generation:

Wood generates fire: liver-blood nourishes mind.

Fire generates earth: heart-yang warms and activates spleen-yang. (in *Internal Classic*, it is considered that heart-fire is source of the human body's yang-qi, while later generations think that kidney-fire is the root of man's yang-qi, and then it is believed that kidney-yang warms and activates spleen-yang.)

Earth generates metal: spleen-qi releases vital essence which gathers in lung to nourish lung-qi.

Metal generates water: lung-qi is purifying and descending, dredging and regulating water passages to help kidney-qi circulate water.

Water generates wood: kidney-yin nourishes liver-yin, that is, water can moisten wood.

Clarifying restrictive relation between five internal organs with five-element restriction:

Wood restricts earth: liver-qi scatters freely to dredges spleen-qi, which enables transportation and transformation of spleen-qi.

Water restricts fire: kidney-water ascends to heart in order to restrain heart-fire from flaming up, which contributes to coordination of water and fire.

Earth restricts water: spleen-qi transports and transforms to help kidney-qi circulate water.

Fire restricts metal: heart-yang is warm, which restrains lung-metal from being excessively pure and descending.

Metal restricts wood: lung-qi is purifying and descending, which restrains liver-qi from sending up excessively.

Mutual help and restriction between five internal organs preserve their balance and coordination as well as normal vital functions of the human body.

③Establishing demic physiological system. Five-element theory classifies human tissues, structures, viscera, organs, physiological functions and vital phenomena into five elements and forms five physiological systems centered by five internal organs. Besides, it clarifies connections of five internal organs' functions with five-element mutual relation and applies five internal organs to unify the human body, which integrates the human body as an organic whole.

Table of Demic Physiological System

Elements	Internal organs	Fu-organs	Body constituents	Sense organs	Mentations	Emotions	Humors	Honors	Meridians
wood	liver	gall-bladder	tendons	eyes	soul	anger	tear	claw	wiry
fire	heart	small intestine	vessel	tongue	mind	joy	sweat	complexion	full
earth	spleen	stomach	muscle	mouth intention	miss	mucus	lips	slow	metal
metal	lung	large intestine	hair	nose	vigor	sadness	nasal discharge	body hair	floating
water	kidney	sanjiao	bones	ears, two lower orifices	will	fear	saliva	hair	deep

The human physiological system based on five-element theory is

223

centered by five internal organs. Every constituent of a system acts under the command of the organ. The functions of six fu-organs, body shape, five sense organs, five humors, five honors, and so on all rely on five internal organs. For example, gallbladder relies on liver-qi to dredge; small intestine relies on heart-yang to warm; stomach relies on spleen-qi to ascend clear; large intestine relies on lung-qi to purify and descend; bladder and sanjiao relies kidney qi to evaporate, and so on; some are presentation of physiological function of five internal organs, such as five mentations, five emotions, five honors, five meridians, and so on.

Human physiological system based on five-element theory further establishes the concept that man is an integrated and organic whole.

(3) Establishing pathological theory

①Etiological theory. According to the uniform relation based on five-element theory, it is proposed that wind invades liver, heat invades heart, dampness invades spleen, dryness invades lung and cold invades kidney. In a similar way, it is inferred that diseases in liver usually present syndrome of stirring wind; diseases in heart usually present heat syndrome; diseases in spleen often present syndrome of damp obstruction; diseases in lung often impair humors and present dry syndrome, and diseases in kidney occur usually due to cold.

②Establishing theory of progress of five internal organs' diseases. It is put forward according to the relation of five-element generation, restriction, supervision and transformation. The progress of five

224

internal organs' diseases can develop in the direction of mutual generation or mutual restriction. In the direction of mutual generation, diseases spread from mother-organs to child-organs, which is called mother-organ disorder involves its child-organs. For example, kidney is water-organ, liver is wood-organ and water can generate wood, so kidney is mother-organ and liver is child-organ. If shortage of kidney-essence appears in the beginning, it will further cause loss of liver-blood and lead to loss of blood and essence in both liver and kidney; or if shortage of kidney-water appears in the beginning and liver-wood cannot get nourishment, then it will cause deficiency of yin in both liver and kidney and excess of liver-yang, which is also believed water fails to nourish wood. All these belong to "mother-organ disorder involves child-organ". In *Difficult Classic*, this progress method is called indirect progress, and "progress leads to generation" is put forward. It is considered that diseases progress in this way always have a favorable prognosis.

If diseases in child-organ affect mother-organ, it is called child steals mother's qi. Heart is fire-organ, and liver is wood-organ. Wood can make fire, so liver is mother-organ and heart is child organ. If there are excessive anxiety and stress, it consumes heart-blood unconsciously, impairs liver and causes loss of liver-blood, and finally gives rise to deficiency of heart and liver blood ; or if heart-fire flames up in the beginning and compromises liver, it will lead to hyperactivity of heart-liver fire. These all belong to "child-organ disorder involves

225

mother-organ" or "child steals mother's qi".

If the progress of five internal organs' diseases develops in the direction of mutual restriction, i. e., mutual invasion, then emotional upset will restrain liver-qi and lead to its stagnation, then transverse invasion in spleen-earth will stop spleen from transportation and transformation, which is called liver-qi invading spleen, also "wood restricting earth". Deficiency of spleen-qi will weaken spleen-yang and prompts spleen to absorb kidney-yang, which leads to deficiency of spleen-kidney yang; if heart-fire flames up, after a long time, it will consume lung-yin and lead to syndrome of deficiency of yin and hyperactivity of fire in heart and lung. These all are the progress in the direction of mutual restriction, called mutual invasion. In *Difficult Classic*, it is called seven progresses of diseases, and also "seven progresses of diseases lead to death" is proposed, which means that if the progress of diseases is in this way, the prognosis is unfavorable.

If the pathological progress develops in the opposite direction of mutual restriction, it is called mutual insult, inverse insult, or inverse restriction. If overeating causes obstruction of spleen-qi and involves liver in, then liver-qi is restrained, which will lead to obstruction of earth and stagnation of wood. If heart-yang is deficient, kidney-yang will be taken away and become deficient, then water will no longer be restrained, which finally gives rise to extreme excess of yin-cold——syndrome of water attacking heart. If liver-fire is excessive, yin-fluid is consumed. After a long time, it will exert bad effect on lung, impair

226

lung-yin, and lead to wood-fire impairing metal. These are symptoms of mutual insult.

To learn progress of five internal organs' diseases by five-element generation and restriction has certain clinical meaning. Clinically common diseases such as liver-qi attacking stomach, wood-fire impairing metal, water-qi attacking heart, water-qi attacking lung, obstruction of earth and stagnation of wood, deficiency of heart and spleen, deficiency of spleen and kidney, deficiency of liver-yin and kidney-yin, heart-kidney imbalance and so on are all related to five-element generation and restriction. However, the progress of diseases are complicated. In *Su Wen · Yu Ji Zhen Zang Lun*, it is said that if diseases happen in sudden, it is not necessarily to treat the viscera to which the diseases will develop according to the progress. In other words, the progress may not develop in light of the sequence of five-element generation and restriction. It means that it may be valuable to learn progress of five internal organs' diseases according to five-element generation and restriction , but it is not the only progressing pattern, so it should be treated flexibly.

(4) Providing theoretical bases for TCM Diagnostics

In *Ling Shu · Ben Zang*, it is said that to diagnose the corresponding part of internal organs on body surface can help learn their condition and diseases. Man is an organic whole, and the diseases inside the body will necessarily reflect in the body surface.

When internal organs are in disorder, it will cause the changes of their physiological functions and mutual relations with relevant organs, which can be reflected in body surface and result in changes of colors, sounds, forms, gustation, pulse condition, and so on. In *Difficult Classic*, it is said that those who learn state of illness by observation treat it in light of five colors; those who learn state of illness by listening treat it based on five tones; those who learn state of illness by asking treat it on the basis of the patient's favor of five flavors; those who learn state of illness by taking the pulse will feel the patient's Cunkou pulse to distinguish whether it is feeble or forceful and locate the organs where diseases happen. The diagnostic approaches of TCM mentioned here are observation, listening, asking and pulse taking, called four methods of diagnosis.

Clinical symptoms that are summarized by four diagnostic methods can be classified into five internal organs according to five-element theory, so as to judge the location and extent of diseases. The diagnostic bases are changes of clinical manifestation in colors, gustation, pulse condition and so on, which are categorized into five internal organs.

Table of Five Internal Organs's Pathological Progress

Elements	Internal organs diseases	Consumption	Colors	Flavors	Body constituents	Sense organs	Pulse condition	Symptoms
wood	liver disease	long-time walking hurts tendons	green	sour	tendon contracture	blurry eyes	wiry	propping fullness in ribs
fire	heart disease	long-time watching impairs blood	red	bitter	vessel stagnation	red tongue	full	distracted
earth	spleen disease	long-time sitting hurts flesh	yellow	sweet	loss flesh	greasy mouth	slow, moderate	abdominal distension, poor appetite
metal	lung disease	long-time lying impairs qi	white	pungent	dryness hair	nasal congestion	floating	cough and asthma, shortness of breath
water	kidney disease	long-time standing hurts bones	black	salty	atrophic debility of bones	deafness	deep	coma, lumbago and faint limb legs

If the symptoms are blue complexion, acidophilic, wiry pulse, and so on, then it is hepatopathy; if they are red complexion, bitter taste, full pulse and so on, then it is heart disease. It is according to the relation between clinical manifestation and viscera that practitioners the location of diseases.

If they are spleen and stomach diseases, the symptoms are yellow complexion, soft and moderate pulse. If the complexion is blue or pulse is wiry, it is liver invading spleen. If it is heart disease, then the complexion is red and pulse is full and rapid. If complexion is dark and pulse is deep, weak, thready and rapid, this is sign of water restricting fire, i. e. , water-qi attacking heart. According to occurrence of different symptoms in the clinical ones, practitioners judge the changes of diseases and the relationship among viscera in disease.

(5) Establishing theory of TCM therapeutics

In clinical treatment, it has to regulate the function of viscera and their mutual relation according to the theory of five-element generation, restriction, supervision and transformation.

In *Difficult Classic*, it is said that if it has been learned that the disease is in liver, then it should be aware that it is prone to affect spleen, so spleen-qi should be tonified first. This is the application of preventing diseases before onset that is proposed in *Internal Classics*.

The treatment of deficiency and excess syndrome can be regulated in light of five-element generation, restriction, supervision and transformation. According to "mother can nourish child" and " child relies on mother's qi", the basic principle for treating deficiency and excess syndromes is that if it is deficiercy, then tonify mother, and if it is syndromes, purge child. For deficiency syndromes, it can be treated through tonifying mother-organ to restore the disordered organ; for excess syndromes, it can be treated through purging child-organ to purge the disordered organ. "Reinforcing earth to generate metal" is a common approach to treat deficiency syndromes of lung. According to the relation of earth generating metal, to tonify spleen-qi is to tonify lung. Under the condition of excessive liver-fire, since fire is son of

230

wood, to purge heart-fire is to purge liver-fire.

There are therapeutic rules based on five-element generation, such as enriching water to nourish wood, tonifying fire to complement earth, reinforcing earth to generate metal, mutual generation between metal and water, and so on; also there are rules proposed in light of five-element restriction, such as reinforcing earth to reduce wood, reinforcing earth to restrain water, assisting metal to calm wood, reducing the south to reinforce the north, and so on.

In acupuncture, these rules can be applied to guide the therapy.

(6) Application in TCP

Application of five-element theory in TCP is mainly to summarize drug effects and their relation with five internal organs.

Five flavors refer to flavors of medicines which can be divided into sour, bitter, sweet, pungent and salty. They have different effects. In *Su Wen · Zang Qi Fa Shi Lun*, it is said that pungent medicines have the effect of divergence, and they are usually used to diverge wind-cold or regulate qi; sour medicines have the effects of astringency and promoting production of body humors, which can be used to astringe body humors and qi, strengthen the intestines for antidiarrheal and quench; bitter medicines have the effects of consolidating yin, purging fire, eliminating dampness and removing heat, so they can be used in the conditions of unconsolidation of kidney-qi, excess of fire-toxin, excess of both dampness and heat and stagnation of fu-qi; salty medicines have the effects of softening hardness to dissipate stagnation as well as moistening dryness and storing body hu-

231

mors, so they can be applied in the occasions of abdominal mass and agglomeration, swellings, consumption of yin-fluid. Five flavors are one of the bases for drug use.

According to five-element theory, five flavors also have relation with five internal organs. In *Su Wen · Zhi Zhen Yao Da Lun*, it is said: "sour first enters liver, bitter first enters heart, sweet first enters spleen, pungent first enters lung, and salty flavor first enters kidney." It indicates that after five flavors enter the human body, each has its own destination. Therefore, they can not only tonify but also impair internal organs. For example, medicines of sour flavor can tonify liver, but if excessive, they can impair liver too.

4. Yin-yang theory and five-element theory

Yin-yang theory and five-element theory were originally two philosophical theories in ancient China, and merged as yin-yang and five elements theory in the end of Warring States period. The yin-yang and five elements theory from TCM theory is mainly the merged version.

Yin-yang theory and five-element theory have been introduced earlier. They both are ancient naive materialism and dialectics thoughts. They have similar and different points.

(1) The common points of yin-yang theory and five-element theory

①Both are Chinese ancient naive materialism and dialectics thoughts.

②Both explain a relatively independent whole and the maintenance of its interior stability.

③Both adopt analogy to classify and apply isomorphic theory to learn matters or phenomena.

④Both are based on the balance theory. They explain stable state of things with balance and coordination, describe relating ways with mutual generation and restriction, and use self-regulating system that consists of the two relating ways to preserve the inner balance and coordination, as well as things' movement, development and changes.

⑤Yin-yang and five elements are abstract and relative concepts. They do not refer to specific matters or phenomena, but have prescription on attributes.

⑥Both take generation and restriction that exceed normality as abnormality or pathological phenomena.

(2) Mutual complementation of yin-yang theory and five-element theory

①"Two" is the cardinal number in yin-yang theory. In mathematics, it is binary system, and in methodology, it is dichotomy. "Five" is the cardinal number in five-element theory. In mathematics, it is decimal system, and in methodology it is polytomy.

②In terms of methods of maintaining interior balance and coordination of matters, yin-yang theory applies direct negative feedback, while five-element theory adopts indirect negative feedback.

③Yin-yang and five elements theory uses the methods of dividing of five elements in yin-yang and dividing yin and yang in five elements to merge yin-yang theory and five-element theory together and take use of them. In TCM theory, when physiological and pathological phenomena are analyzed, it has the division of both five internal organs and yin-yang, i. e. , division of yin-yang in five internal organs (every internal organ involves yin and yang, qi and blood), and division of five internal organs in yin-yang (the human body has division of yin-yang, yin involves five internal organs, and yang involves five fu-organs).